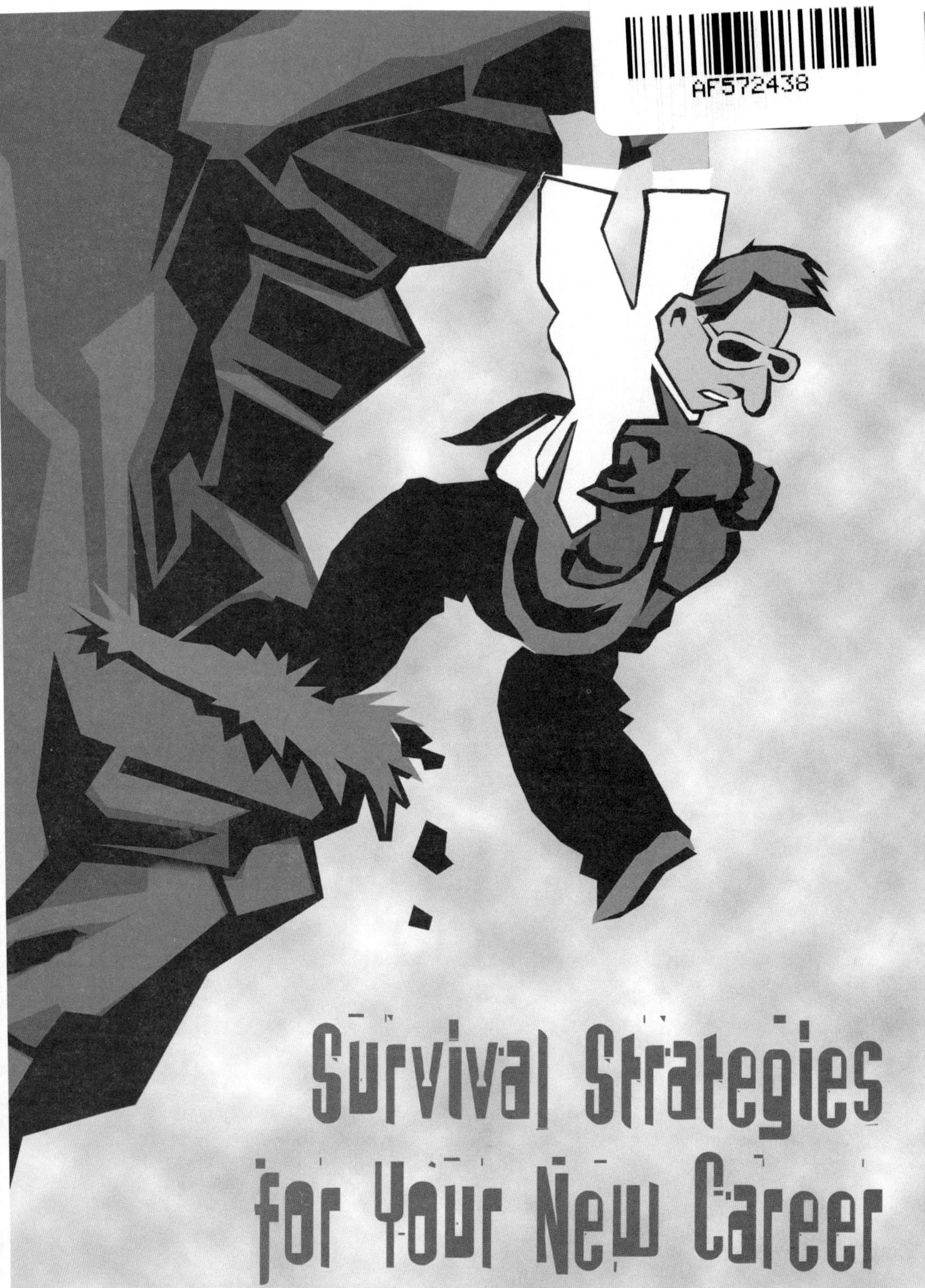

Survival Strategies for Your New Career

American Society of Health-System Pharmacists®

Published by the American Society of Health-System Pharmacists, 7272 Wisconsin Avenue, Bethesda, MD 20814.

Clip content adapted from TASK FORCE ImageGALLERY, NVTech Inc.

ISBN: 1-58528-031-3

Table of Contents

**Note:* Practitioners spotlighted here may have changed positions or offices since the manuscript was prepared.

Authors, Contributors, and Reviewers

Authors

David M. Reile, Ph.D., NCCC
Jill L. Nickols, Pharm.D., M.B.A.

Contributors

Keri A. Mattes, Pharm.D.
Brian Cohen, Pharm.D.
Dianne E. Tobias, Pharm.D.
Jan Allen, R.Ph., FASCP
Cynthia Brennan, Pharm.D., M.H.A.
Helen S. Yee, Pharm.D.
Rita K. Jew, Pharm.D.
Marianne Billeter, Pharm.D., BCPS
Burnis D. Breland, Pharm.D., M.S.
Keith M. Olsen, Pharm.D., FCCP
Kent M. Nelson, Pharm.D., BCPS
Darlene M. Mednick, M.B.A., R.Ph., PAHN, NPDP
Jane S. Henry, M.B.A., R.Ph., FASHP
Joseph T. Botticelli, M.S., R.Ph.
Stanley N. Chamallas, R.Ph., FASHP
Donald J. Filibeck, Pharm.D., M.B.A.

Reviewers

Bruce A. Nelson, M.S., R.Ph.
Jill L. Nickols, Pharm.D., M.B.A.
Hannah J. Kim, Pharm.D.
John Michael O'Brien, Pharm.D.
Martha Davies

Welcome from the American Society of Health-System Pharmacists

You have embarked upon an important career. As a health-system pharmacist, you will impact the lives and health of many people. Patients, their families, nurses, and physicians will rely on you, your knowledge, and your expertise. You are an integral part of the medical community. As you move forward, the American Society of Health-System Pharmacists (ASHP) wants you to know that you are not alone. Membership in ASHP has many benefits, including advice and support in your career development. You may be comfortable and confident in your current work setting. Or perhaps you have not quite found your niche. Whether you feel established, are still looking, or want to keep your options open for the future, ASHP's *Survival Strategies for Your New Career* is filled with information and helpful tips to aid you in your practice of health-system pharmacy.

We wish you much success.

Henri R. Manasse, Jr., Ph.D., Sc.D.

An Introduction to Health-System Pharmacy . . .

Health-system pharmacy spans a broad spectrum of pharmacy practice. It includes working in hospitals, long-term-care facilities, health maintenance and home care organizations, and ambulatory care clinics. These settings typically allow pharmacists to work closely with physicians, nurses, and other health care professionals in medication therapy management, clinical laboratory evaluation, patient counseling, and general patient care. A health-system pharmacist is considered an expert in drug information and interpretation by these interdisciplinary teams. A pharmacist is also the source of prescription distribution, ensuring that patients receive the appropriate medication in a safe and timely manner.

Many pharmacists find the real world of pharmacy practice different than they imagined while in school. In the classroom, their future in pharmacy practice seemed full of promise and endless possibilities. It seemed to offer the opportunity to get to know patients and make a significant impact on their health, while working cooperatively with other medical professionals and integrating comprehensive pharmaceutical care into daily activities. However, once they are licensed and practicing, some forget the ideal practice model they once envisioned and struggle simply to complete necessary daily responsibilities, such as filling orders and dispensing medication. The reality of the daily routine may overwhelm the desire to provide complete and effective pharmaceutical care. However, pharmacists working in a health system can find an opportunity to provide quality direct care to patients.

A health-system pharmacist provides accurate information to the patient and health care team, as well as conducts research and quality checks to detect and avoid possible drug interactions, adverse effects, and medication errors. Health-system pharmacists work with other medical professionals and patients to achieve the best possible health care outcome. These pharmacists are responsible for counseling patients and their families on proper medication usage. They maintain open communication with patients about concerns they might have about medication therapy, previous and concomitant health conditions, and other crucial information that might affect a patient's medication therapy compliance. The pharmacist assesses a patient's understanding of his or her medication therapy to ensure both the patient and health care providers are working together to achieve positive patient outcomes.

Health-system pharmacists are highly educated professionals with a minimum of five years of pharmacy education. As the Doctor of Pharmacy (Pharm.D.) becomes the entry-level degree across the nation, the current minimum of five years of training is increasing to six or more. More and more pharmacy graduates also complete residency or fellowship training lasting at least one year. Some pharmacists are opting for additional training to specialize in particular pharmacy practice areas, such as geriatrics, pediatrics, oncology, cardiology, infectious diseases, pharmacokinetics, or critical care. Postgraduate residency training provides practitioners with the knowledge and experience needed to face the evolving challenges in health-system pharmacy practice and emphasizes essential skills needed to meet practice demands. Residency and fellowship training are discussed further in chapter 2.

The possible career avenues available to a health-system pharmacist are numerous. One might opt to practice in a variety of settings, such as ambulatory care clinics, home infusion companies, long-term-care facilities, managed care organizations, and hospitals. Responsibilities in these settings differ considerably, from preparing sterile injectable medications to making rounds on hospital floors to serving as an administrator who coordinates budget allocations and represents the pharmacy department to the organization. The roles available to a health-system pharmacist depend on his or her personal preferences and the type of activities and personal interactions desired.

We have spotlighted eight areas to showcase some of the opportunities that exist. Throughout the book you will find the profiles of several practitioners who will share with you information about their academic backgrounds, past and current work experiences, and their involvement with pharmacy associations. Also, those who have hiring responsibilities let us know what they look for in a job applicant.

Chapter 1

Choosing and Changing Careers

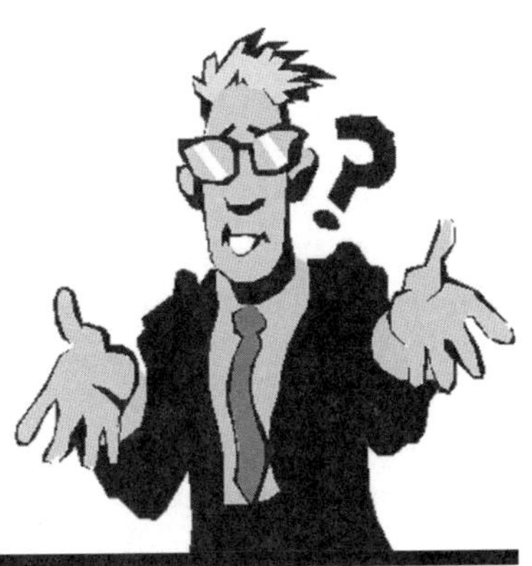

Finding a Job You Enjoy

You've chosen a career in pharmacy—more specifically, health-system pharmacy. Within health-system pharmacy you have learned that you have many career options to choose from, anything from working in a hospital clinical setting to home care to teaching to managing other pharmacists. You can see from the career summaries interspersed throughout the book that moving from one practice setting to another is common and may allow for upward career mobility that might not exist for an individual health-system pharmacist in one job setting.

It is expected that in a typical forty-year career as a health-system pharmacist, you will spend over 100,000 hours on the job. That's more time than you will spend in any other single activity—for many this may even include time spent sleeping! If you are going to spend this much time working, it needs to be doing something you enjoy in an environment that you find pleasing. The obvious question for many then is, "How do I do this?"

Understanding yourself is key to finding a job you enjoy. In career planning, there are five areas most frequently considered vital: values, interests, skills, work environment and compensation factors, and personality. Interests and skills assessment doesn't end when you become a pharmacist in a health system. Determining what practice setting is right for you now and in the future will be aided greatly if you take the time to consider the following work-life factors.

Values. Values provide motivation and meaning in our lives and include concepts like spending time with family, being honest, having integrity, being an authority in your field, and earning a good living. In doing a review of your values, consider what is most important to you in the following areas of life:

- relationships
- finances
- career/work
- education/learning
- spirituality/ethics/morality
- physical health
- mental health, and
- personal time.

Think about each of these areas, and write out statements that describe the elements of these that are most important to you. Use the worksheets on pages 16 and 17 to help examine your values. When you have completed this exercise, please list your top three values and record them on the summary sheet on page 23.

Interests. Interests are the things we enjoy doing. Think about what you enjoy most about your work as a health-system pharmacist. Think about all aspects of your day. Do you enjoy working one-on-one with patients or teaching pharmacy students or planning the annual budget? Use the worksheet on page 18 to help examine your interests. Once you have completed this exercise, please select your top three interests and record them on your summary sheet on page 23.

Skills. Skills are the abilities we count as our strengths. Think very carefully about what you do well. In addition to your clinical pharmacy skills, think about other skills that you possess, such as interpersonal, teaching, and organizational abilities. Also, try to connect your core skills with your interests. Skills that you enjoy doing are more useful to you than skills you prefer not to use. One way to assess your skills is to think about times in your life when you have been the most successful. The worksheet on page 19 will guide you through a skills assessment exercise. When you have completed this activity, name your top three skills on the summary sheet on page 24.

Work Environment and Compensation Factors. Work environment and items related to compensation are among the elements that influence on-the-job satisfaction. These include such things as commute time, whether you work alone or with a team, how much supervision you give or receive, and whether you have an office. Think about a typical day or week of work. Use the worksheet on pages 21 and 22 to help examine your work environment preferences. When you have completed this exercise, record your top work environment preferences on the summary sheet on page 24.

Work-Life Factors Summary

Using the Work-Life Factors Summary on pages 23 and 24, review the values, interests, skills, and work environment preferences that are most important to you. To what degree are these factors satisfied in your daily work? Review the work-life satisfaction grid and rate your current level of on-the-job satisfaction on each of these factors and your current overall level of satisfaction. When you have determined the degree to which your current work satisfies your values, interests, skills, and environmental factors, you need to compare this to the other career options.

Next Steps

Understanding your current level of job satisfaction is the first step in evaluating your career options. The next step is to determine what other options are available to you and the degree to which these may increase or decrease your current level of satisfaction.

Knowledge of your other career options may begin with a book like this one. Read through career summaries in this book. Which ones seem appealing to you? Contact ASHP and get the name of someone in your area who is practicing in a specialty of interest to you. Conduct an informational interview with this person and ask questions that will help you determine the match between this other career specialty and your work-life factors preferences.

An informational interview is a meeting to learn more about a health-system pharmacy specialty from a pharmacist who works in this area. It is often a good idea to conduct more than one informational interview for each specialty of interest in order to get a well-rounded perspective and hear several points of view.

As you are the interviewer, it is important that you know in advance what you hope to gain from the interview and that you plan accordingly. A list of suggested questions to ask in informational interviews is on pages 25 and 26. You should also think of questions unique to your Work-Life Factors Summary.

Residency Training

Having spent some time in self-assessment and conducting informational interviews, you may have begun to wonder if a residency is right for you. Pharmacy residencies began in the early 1930s as internships to train pharmacists in hospital pharmacy management. Today, ASHP has developed accreditation standards recognizing seventeen specialty areas and has recently formed partnerships with other pharmacy associations (e.g., Academy of Managed Care Pharmacy, American College of Clinical Pharmacy, American Pharmaceutical Association [APhA], and the American Society of Consultant Pharmacists) for joint accreditation of residencies. Currently there are 533 accredited and accreditation-pending residency programs (313 pharmacy practice and 220 specialty). The total number of pharmacy practice residency positions available in the recent match was 804.

Residency training can take place in a variety of health-care settings—some of which include hospitals, home care, long-term-care programs, ambulatory care settings, and managed care facilities. The type of residency you select will depend upon your career objectives. Are you interested in providing pharmaceutical care to a broad mix of patients? pursuing a career in pharmacy administration? becoming a specialized practitioner or educator? Based on your interests and experience level, you will need to complete a residency in pharmacy practice or a specialized pharmacy residency, or both.

In addition to preparing pharmacists for practice by exposing them to a wide range of patients, residency training offers several advantages:

- *A competitive advantage in the job market.* More and more employers recognize the value of residency training. A pharmacist who has completed a residency will have a clear advantage over applicants who have not.

- *Networking opportunities.* Many opportunities arise for residents to establish or expand their network of professional acquaintances and contacts, including preceptors and other residents.

New Practitioner

Keri A. Mattes, Pharm.D.

Assistant Professor, St. Louis College of Pharmacy, St. Louis, Missouri

Dr. Keri Mattes teaches courses on pharmacotherapy and women's health. In addition to her didactic responsibilities, Dr. Mattes is a preceptor for clerkship students doing their general medicine rotation. Dr. Mattes' professional responsibilities are not limited to the classroom, however, as she is also a clinician at the St. Louis Veterans Affairs Medical Center. In this role, she is a member of an interdisciplinary inpatient general medicine team and a practitioner in the outpatient infectious disease clinic. During a typical day, Dr. Mattes goes on rounds with the medicine team, recommends drug selections, monitors drug therapy, educates the medicine team about pertinent pharmacotherapy issues, and educates patients about their drug therapy.

Dr. Mattes graduated with a Pharm.D. degree from the University of Iowa in 1999. Through her involvement with ASHP as a student, she was exposed to a variety of internships and networking opportunities, including an adult internal medicine residency at Family Medicine of St. Louis. During her residency, she gained experience in clinical pharmacy and teaching.

Dr. Mattes credits her active involvement with ASHP on local and national levels as a strong contributor to her professional development. While at the University of Iowa, she served as the president of the local student health-system pharmacy society and took on a national role as the chair of the ASHP Student Forum Executive Committee. As chair, she performed outreach visits to colleges of pharmacy, participated as an observer in ASHP Board of Directors meetings, and contributed to the development of student programming at ASHP national meetings. These activities helped her to develop leadership, planning, and communication skills, and she feels the networking opportunities she had as a result of her ASHP duties were key to her obtaining a residency and a job.

She has continued this involvement with ASHP in her professional practice and currently serves as the faculty advisor of the St. Louis College of Pharmacy student society. She assists students in defining and achieving their career goals. Dr. Mattes contends, "ASHP has opened many doors for me, and I continue to learn from people that I've met through my membership and involvement in the organization." The advice Dr. Mattes offers to new practitioners is to continue to pursue opportunities that allow you to grow and learn.

- *Career planning.* During the course of training, most residents gain a clearer picture of what type of practice best suits them. Residency preceptors are committed to providing personal attention and assisting each resident in further defining professional goals.

- *Professional vision.* Many programs also offer the opportunity to see how pharmacy is practiced in different parts of the country by arranging for residents to visit other residency programs or by allowing residents to complete a portion of the residency at another site (e.g., acute care, community care, home care, long-term care, managed care, etc.).

Specialized Pharmacy Residencies. ASHP recognizes specialized residencies in an ever expanding number of areas: cardiology, clinical pharmacokinetics, critical care, drug information, emergency medicine, geriatrics, infectious diseases, internal medicine, managed care pharmacy systems, nuclear pharmacy, nutrition support, oncology, pediatrics, pharmacotherapy, pharmacy practice management, primary care, and psychiatric pharmacy practice.

A specialized pharmacy residency is designed to build upon competencies developed by a residency in pharmacy practice. All ASHP-accredited residencies are full-time commitments that require at least one year to complete. Because many specialty residencies require that the applicant have completed a pharmacy practice residency, one should plan for two years of training after receiving an academic degree. Some specialized residencies may be offered in combination with other programs, such as a fellowship, which may require additional years to complete.

Requirements for Residency Admission

1) You must be a graduate of an ACPE-accredited college of pharmacy or otherwise be eligible for licensure.

2) You will need to demonstrate your interest in and aptitude for advanced training in pharmacy.

3) Some residencies require that you be licensed to practice before you enter the program. Others will accept you while you pursue state board licensure.

4) For residencies that are combined with a graduate degree program, you must satisfy the requirements of the college of pharmacy or gradu-

New Practitioner

Brian Cohen, Pharm.D.

Second Year Pharmacy Practice Management Resident, University of Kansas Medical Center

Dr. Brian Cohen is a 1999 graduate of the University of Texas at Austin. Before becoming a licensed pharmacist, he worked as a pharmacy technician for six years. He served as an administrative resident at the University of Kansas Medical Center. Among his many duties, he participated in all pharmacy and therapeutics committee activities, maintained departmental statistics, managed student interns, implemented departmental medication safety initiatives, and developed Web pages. During his various residency rotations he had the opportunity to participate in and learn general practice skills, surgical trauma, drug information and drug policy, investigational drug services, operating room pharmacy, inpatient and outpatient infectious disease, organizational improvement, association management with ASHP, medication safety, financial management, and database and Web page development.

Dr. Cohen says, "ASHP has had a large impact on my professional development. [It has] encouraged me to pursue a residency, enhanced my leadership skills, provided the opportunity for me to get involved at all levels of organizational management, and exposed me to national pharmacy practice." Dr. Cohen has been an active participant in pharmacy organizations, serving in leadership positions at school, state, and national levels. He was president of the University of Texas Student Society of Health-System Pharmacists and the first chair of the student section of the Texas Society of Health-System Pharmacists. On the national level, Dr. Cohen is a past member of the ASHP Student Forum Executive Committee and a past chair of the ASHP Student Forum Programming Committee.

Regarding advice to a new practitioner, Dr. Cohen says, "Do a residency! Residencies provide unique opportunities to explore different aspects of pharmacy as a licensed practitioner. No other [training] allows a pharmacist to gain vast amounts of experience in such a short period of time. Also, stay involved with pharmacy organizations as a new practitioner. Pharmacy organizations are essential to securing pharmacy's role on the health care team."

ate school for admission to the advanced degree program. In addition, you will need to satisfy the residency requirements.

5) Residents in ASHP-accredited programs are encouraged to be members of ASHP.

There are some additional qualifications for a residency, such as excellent written and oral communication skills, organizational and time management skills, leadership ability, good decision-making skills, and participation in both professional and social organizations.

For more information about ASHP-accredited residencies, contact

Accreditation Services Division
ASHP
7272 Wisconsin Avenue
Bethesda, MD 20814
Phone: (301) 657-3000, ext. 1251
Fax: (301) 664-8867
asd@ashp.org

The Resident Matching Program. ASHP contracts with the National Matching Service (NMS) to operate a Resident Matching Program for residencies in pharmacy practice. The Matching Program ensures that each pharmacy practice residency program will be matched with the preferred individuals who have applied and who have selected the program as an acceptable site in which to train. To apply for an ASHP-accredited pharmacy practice residency, you must sign up for the Resident Matching Program. Contact NMS for information and an applicant agreement form that serves as your enrollment. NMS must receive your agreement form and your enrollment form and fee by January 15 of each year to be considered for a residency beginning that year.

Once you have enrolled with NMS, you should access the ASHP Residency Directory on the ASHP website at www.ashp.org. In it you'll find descriptions of all accredited residencies, along with important contact information. (Note: ASHP-accredited specialized residencies do not participate in the Matching Program; however, most specialized residency programs require that you have completed a residency in pharmacy practice before applying for a specialized residency.)

After consulting the Residency Directory and identifying programs of interest, you will need to request application forms from individual pro-

Practitioner Spotlight

Ambulatory Care

Cynthia Brennan, Pharm.D., M.H.A.

Assistant Director, Harborview Medical Center Pharmacy
Associate Clinical Professor, University of Washington School of Pharmacy
Director, Primary Care Specialty Residency Program, University of Washington Academic Medical Centers

Dr. Cynthia Brennan balances a multitude of professional pharmacy roles. She has served since 1990 in her current capacity as assistant director for the Harborview Medical Center Pharmacy, where she is accountable for a $14 million drug budget and 72 full-time pharmacists and technicians. She is responsible for strategic planning for pharmaceutical care services in the ambulatory care clinics at Harborview. She connects pharmacy practitioners to various programs within and outside of her institution and provides them with the resources and support they need to succeed.

Dr. Brennan attends a number of multidisciplinary meetings that include care providers and administrators. She works on program development, utilization management, quality improvement, workload and outcomes tracking, and personnel issues. She also works with the assistant director of inpatient pharmacy to coordinate pharmaceutical care across the continuum.

Dr. Brennan began working for Harborview in 1980 after graduation from the University of Southern California School of Pharmacy with a Pharm.D. degree. After a year on the trauma surgery team, she was offered a newly created position as the pharmacist on the critical care team. During this time, Dr. Brennan developed an expertise in cardiology and began to teach sections in cardiology at the University of Washington School of Pharmacy. In 1986, an ambulatory supervisor position was created at Harborview, and Dr. Brennan was selected. The Harborview HIV/AIDS clinic was just beginning to use zidovidine treatment, and Dr. Brennan was asked to manage this new drug. This opportunity led to the development of an additional area of expertise. Dr. Brennan presented her work at national and international conferences and added this specialty to her teaching at the University of Washington. Dr. Brennan continued to split her time between clinical practice and administrative duties but ultimately had to choose. She was promoted to assistant director of ambulatory pharmacy services in 1990 and moved out of a clinical role in 1995.

Dr. Brennan has been an active member of ASHP, as well as state and local affiliate chapters, since the beginning of her career. In 1998, she was

continued next page

Cynthia Brennan, Pharm.D., M.H.A. *(continued)*

selected to attend the ASHP/University of North Carolina Leadership Development Institute for pharmacy managers and leaders. This week-long training included leadership development and high-level discussions with colleagues regarding the direction of the pharmacy profession. Also in 1998, Dr. Brennan was selected to serve on ASHP's Council on Administrative Affairs (COAA), one of the five professional policy development councils convened each year at ASHP. The COAA discussed several issues raised by the membership concerning the management of pharmacy resources and the quality of pharmacy services.

Dr. Brennan attributes her broad knowledge of pharmacy practice and her skills in performing clinical and administrative work, as well as her network of colleagues and collaborators, to her involvement in professional organization activities. She expressed, "National involvement helps me place the profession in the context of the greater health care world and helps to refocus my efforts in the development of the profession." For example, in January 2000, Dr. Brennan and her team at Harborview requested approval from the Washington State Board of Pharmacy for full prescriptive authority for clinical pharmacists on the basis of standards of practice and recognized treatment guidelines. Primary care pharmacists needed the flexibility to treat patients with multiple chronic conditions, and strict disease-based protocols were deemed too rigid. The state board approved this flexible prescriptive authority provided that quarterly patient outcome reports be sent to them for review.

As an administrator, Dr. Brennan sometimes hires new practitioners. During the course of the interview, she looks for evidence of the ability to learn. Typically, a pharmacist who has completed a pharmacy practice residency and a specialty residency has demonstrated this ability, as well as a commitment to the profession. She also looks for someone with a positive "can do" attitude who can work with pharmacists as well as other health care providers. She likes to see someone who is involved in life beyond pharmacy.

Dr. Brennan offers the following advice to new practitioners, "Commit yourself to lifetime learning; take opportunities to stretch beyond your comfort zone; cherish the trust your patients place in you; and balance your professional and personal life."

grams directors, not from ASHP. Most programs require that you visit the site to complete the application process; however, application procedures vary by program.

The residency programs participating in the Resident Matching Program take part in the ASHP Midyear Clinical Meeting Residency Showcase.

The Residency Showcase, discussed further in chapter 5 (page 88), gives potential applicants the opportunity to meet the current residents, preceptors, and program directors.

For more information about the Resident Match Program, contact

National Matching Services, Inc.
595 Bay Street, Suite 300
Toronto, Ontario
Canada M5G 2C2
Phone: (416) 977-3431
Fax: (416) 977-5020

Fellowship Training

A fellowship differs from a residency in that it prepares a pharmacist for independent research instead of developing patient care skills. Most residencies last one year and involve several preceptors, while most fellowships last two years and involve only one preceptor.

More specifically, fellowships are designed to train pharmacists to conceptualize, plan, conduct, and report independent research. The program is under the guidance of a researcher–preceptor who offers the fellow an individualized learning experience. That experience gives the fellow the training necessary to conduct collaborative research or to function as a principal investigator. The type of research performed can range from pharmacy policy to drug development to laboratory research.

Pharmacists in fellowship programs may spend some time in patient care but generally spend much less time than residents. Fellows may also have teaching responsibilities in addition to research activities. In selecting a pharmacy fellowship it is important to match your interests to the type of research being conducted by the fellowship preceptor. Participants may be expected to have some prior experience in the research area through practice during school or through a residency. While some programs consider a residency a prerequisite to a fellowship, some industry-sponsored fellowships at academic centers do not require them.

Personnel Placement Service

The Personnel Placement Service (PPS) is a career assistance program offered in conjunction with the ASHP Midyear Clinical Meeting. Participants pay a fee to participate in PPS (in addition to the Midyear registration fee), which features specialty residencies, fellowships, and a variety of other employment positions in academia, health-systems, associations, industry, medical communication companies, and other various pharmacy settings. A Web site is set up for registrants to conduct job placement activities online in advance of the meeting. At the meeting, registrants will have access to an exclusive area to participate in personal interviews. Here's an overview of how PPS operates.

Post a Listing. To participate, simply complete the registration form indicating your preferred practice area, location, start date, and other details. Space is also provided to describe the school you are attending, work experience, pharmacy affiliations (e.g., fraternities, societies), and special skills such as languages or computer expertise (see below for examples).

> *Pharmacy Practice Residency:*
> Pharm.D. conferred in May 1999 (University of Iowa). Interests include primary care/ambulatory care, internal medicine, cardiology. Experience: clinical clerkships in cardiology, family medicine, critical care, infectious disease, community pharmaceutical care; oncology research experience. Four years internship in a community pharmacy. Member: ASHP.

> *Pharmacy Practice Residency:*
> Pharm.D. May 1999 (University of Oklahoma), B.S. Biology (University of Oklahoma). Experience: hospital, community, clinical rotations. Interests: cardiology, oncology, ambulatory care, industry. Memberships (positions held): ASHP (Student Delegate), OSHP (Vice President, Historian), Kappa Psi (Treasurer), PLS (Vice President), APhA-ASP (Student Delegate), NCPA.

PPS registration are available on the ASHP Web site. If you register online, you will login with your customer/member ID and use a credit card to purchase your PPS registration through the ASHP shopping cart. After your transaction has been processed (usually within one minute), you will prepare your own listing directly on the PPS Web site. To register by mail or fax, simply send your registration form and payment to ASHP. ASHP will post your listing on the PPS Web site within 7–10 days and send an e-mail confirmation with directions for reviewing and editing your listing online. Regardless of your registration method, e-mail will be the primary method of communication between PPS registrants and ASHP. Be sure to provide a valid e-mail address.

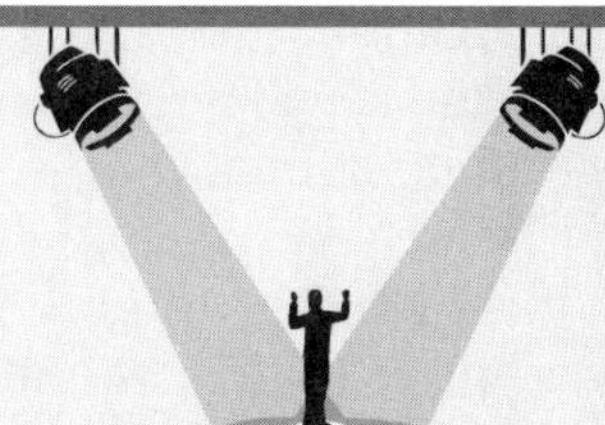

Practitioner Spotlight

Ambulatory Care

Helen S. Yee, Pharm.D.

Ambulatory Care Clinical Pharmacist, Department of Veterans Affairs Medical Center–San Francisco

Dr. Helen Yee has worked as an ambulatory care clinical pharmacist for five years. She provides pharmaceutical care and performs drug-related physical assessments in the anticoagulation, smoking cessation, and pharmaceutical care clinics. She evaluates patient outcomes, assists in staff development, develops patient counseling materials, and conducts research. She is a preceptor for students and residents, teaches, conducts patient education classes, and is responsible for staffing and code blue coverage. She has provided pharmaceutical care and performed drug-related assessments in chest, medical practice (metabolism), neurology, and evaluation and assessment (urgent care) clinics. She implemented a pharmaceutical care clinic and evaluated its impact on outcomes as a research project.

Early in her career, Dr. Yee benefited from a pharmacy practice residency and a primary care specialty residency. She has been involved with local, state, and national pharmacy organizations. Currently, she is a reviewer for the ASHP Ambulatory Care Clinical Skills Program Modules. She was a reviewer for the *ASHP Medication Teaching Manual: The Guide to Patient Drug Information*. She has served as faculty for ASHP physical assessment workshops and has published articles in the *American Journal of Health-System Pharmacy (AJHP)*. Dr. Yee has been active at the ASHP Midyear Clinical Meetings in a variety of functions—presenting management cases, participating in the poster presentations, and serving as a meeting program associate.

Dr. Yee offers the following advice to new practitioners, "Be open-minded, positive, and flexible! Don't place limitations on what a pharmacist is capable of achieving!"

All listings will be posted on the PPS Web site for employers to review prior to the meeting. Listings received before October 15 will also be published in the Advance Listings book (mailed to employers prior to the meeting). Since not all residency programs participate in PPS, you should ask those that interest you whether they will be interviewing at the meeting.

Search Listings. Search for jobs or residency listings by type, practice area, location, salary, and other criteria in early November on the PPS Web site. Listings will be continuously updated on site until November 20. Searching online allows you to view the most up-to-date job listings and tailor your search to select the best prospects for onsite interviews.

Scheduling Interviews. If you see a job you are interested in during your online search, you may contact the employer in advance of the meeting (if telephone number or e-mail is provided in the listing) to express your interest in interviewing. Employers will also be searching the applicant listings and will either contact you with an assigned interview time and location or ask you to sign up for an interview at their assigned interview booth once the meeting begins. (Note: only applicants who are invited to do so may schedule interviews at an employer's interview booth.) For privacy reasons, ASHP does not release employer booth locations during the meeting. Be sure to keep track of your scheduled interviews and the locations of the interview booths.

If the job listing doesn't include any contact information, you can contact the employer onsite through their PPS mailbox. Do not be concerned if you haven't been contacted before the meeting; many employers prefer to schedule interviews once the meeting begins.

At the Meeting. Each applicant and each position will be assigned a unique mail box number (noted at the top of each listing) to facilitate onsite communication. Remember to bring printed copies of all the job listings that interest you to the meeting so you can easily reference the mail box number, contact name, and other details. Only a limited number of display copies of printed listings will be available onsite.

Once the meeting starts, you can contact employers by delivering message forms (with your résumé attached) to their mail boxes to request an interview. For your convenience, message forms will be provided on the PPS Web site to complete in advance of the meeting. Information on preparing for interviews will also be available on the Web site.

The interviews at PPS usually last about 15 to 30 minutes. The format of the interview depends on the type of program for which an applicant is interviewing. Pharmacy practice residency interviews usually consist of program directors using the entire time to talk about their programs. Other residency programs use this interview as a pre-screening tool and may ask some tough questions.

Keep in mind that PPS is only a preliminary interview and it does not guarantee a job, residency, or fellowship. It should be considered a screening tool both for participants and the programs. If you are being considered for a position, you will most likely have to interview at the site at a later date.

In addition to this career assistance program at the Midyear Clinical Meeting, ASHP will be offering year-round online personnel placement service in Fall/Winter 2001. Employers and applicants can post job listings or résumés, search the site for available applicants or job listings, and exchange résumés and job descriptions online. The service can also search the database for you and e-mail listings on a daily or weekly basis. The site is free for ASHP member job seekers.

PPS Tips. For maximum exposure, register by the advance deadline (early October for mail and fax registrations and mid October for online registration). If you plan to purchase your PPS registration online, you will need your ASHP customer/member ID number and password. If you don't know this information, visit www.ashp.org and click on "member login" to look up or request your password. Be sure that you have a valid e-mail address and that your ASHP membership information (mailing address, phone, fax, and e-mail) is up-to-date.

Participation in PPS is limited to those who are registered to attend the Midyear. You can purchase your PPS registration and post your listing before you register for the Midyear or do them both at the same time (but you must be registered for the Midyear before you arrive at the meeting).

Prepare in advance. Log in to the Web site to screen job listings before the meeting. You will need to do this several times as the information is continuously updated until mid November. Be sure to bring your instructions and assigned PPS mail box number with you to the meeting. This will help you avoid standing in lines at the registration desk to confirm information or ask questions.

Bring office supplies (pens, paper, paper clips, stapler, etc.) and plenty of copies of your résumé to attach to message forms. You may also wish to bring your résumé on disk in case you need to make changes at a business center during the meeting.

Bring copies of the job listings that interest you since you will need to reference this information onsite. Only a limited number of display copies of printed listings will be available at the meeting. With over 1,500 PPS registrants, you don't want to waste valuable time waiting in lines to review listings.

Print and bring with you copies of message forms pre-addressed to prospective employers (with your résumé attached). This will allow you to spend your time reviewing late (onsite) listings and scheduling interviews, instead of completing paperwork.

Values Review

Relationships

Example—having a close family unit; having good and loyal friends; being a good parent

Finances

Example—earning a good salary; saving for my retirement; buying anything I want

Career/Work

Example—having a stable job; working for a prestigious organization; having professional independence

Education/Learning

Example—having an opportunity to update my skills; learning new things

Spirituality/Ethics/Morality

Example—being a spiritual person; being a positive influence

___

___

___

Physical Health

Example—being physically active; maintaining good health

___

___

___

Mental Health

Example—knowing myself; having good relationships

___

___

___

Personal Time

Example—having time to myself; doing what I enjoy

___

___

___

Record these on the summary sheet on page 23.

Interests Review

Use the following planner to write out your typical duties during an average workday. Be as specific as you can. Whether you work in shifts (7:00 am–3:00 pm, 3:00 pm–11:00 pm, 11:00 pm–7:00 am) or have a standard schedule (8:00 am–5:00 pm), write in the times that fit your schedule and activities during those times.

Activities

Morning ______________________________

Time ______________________________

____

Afternoon ______________________________

Time ______________________________

____

Evening ______________________________

Time ______________________________

____

Night ______________________________

Time ______________________________

____

Review your work day. What do you enjoy doing most? What energizes you about your work? Write three things that you are interested in, enjoy, and are most energized by.

____

____

____

Record these on the summary sheet on page 23.

Skills Review

Life Highlights. Think about times in your life that have been highlights for you. These can come from any area of life, not just work. For example:

- Planning a family reunion.
- Working cooperatively with a patient to achieve a positive health outcome
- Managing multiple school projects during a busy semester.
- Supervising students at a summer camp.

In a couple of sentences, write down two or three of these life highlights.

Now, choose one of these highlights and describe the life experience in detail. Specify what was involved in the successful completion of this event by answering "Who," "What," "Where," "When," "Why," "How," and "How Much."

Carefully read over what you have written and select the skills you used in this life achievement.

Repeat the previous two steps for each of the life highlights you recorded on page 19.

____

____

____

____

____

____

Review all of the skills you have listed and select your top five—the skills you believe you can use very competently and that you enjoy most of all. Write them down on the following lines and record these on page 24.

____

____

____

____

____

____

Work Environment and Compensation Factors

What is most important to you about your job or what factors would you change if you had a choice? commute time?, health insurance benefits? a window office? diverse coworkers? Use the following headings to consider the work environments and compensation factors that contribute to your on-the-job satisfaction. Review the factors you have written and circle the three that are most important to you and write them on the summary worksheet on page 24.

Company Factors (i.e., company size, reputation, structure)

____

____

Location and Setting (i.e., travel required, geographic location, proximity to home)

____

____

Working Style (i.e., alone, in a group, dress code)

____

____

Physical Aspects (i.e., noise, lighting, temperature, window office)

____

____

Personal Values (i.e., status, coworker characteristics, challenges)

____

____

Supervision (i.e., little, much)

____

____

Compensation (i.e., benefits, leave time, salary level)

____

____

Business Type (i.e., service, retail, government, education)

____

____

Transportation (i.e., parking available, public transportation accessible)

____

____

Other Factors of Your Choosing

____

____

____

____

____

Work-Life Factors Summary

Satisfaction Quotient

Based on your current work, what percentage of your top values, interests, skills, and work environment preferences are satisfied each week?

not at all satisfied | satisfied about half the time | totally satisfied

0% 10 20 30 40 50 60 70 80 90 100%

Values

1) ____________________

2) ____________________

3) ____________________

Interests

1) ____________________

2) ____________________

3) ____________________

Skills

1) ______________________________

2) ______________________________

3) ______________________________

4) ______________________________

5) ______________________________

Work Environment Preferences

1) ______________________________

2) ______________________________

3) ______________________________

Overall Satisfaction Quotient

Based on your current work week, how satisfied are you overall?

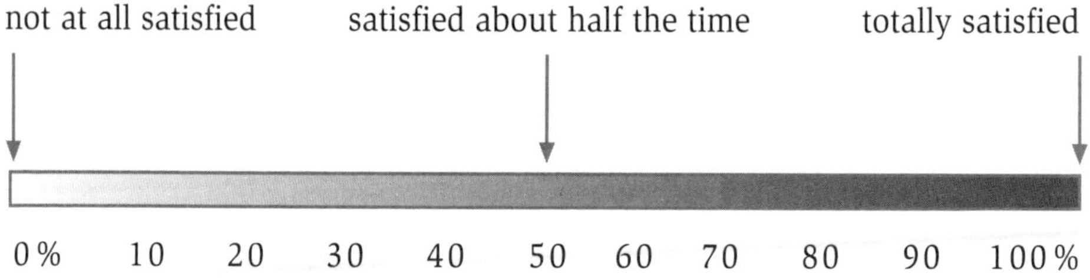

List of Suggested Questions for Informational Interview

1) How and why did you choose this health-system pharmacy specialty?

____

____

2) What do you like most and least about your work?

____

____

3) Are there any residency requirements to work in this field?

____

____

4) What are the various practice settings for this health-system pharmacy specialty?

____

____

5) What are your typical job duties? How do you spend your workday?

____

____

6) What are the salary ranges for new practitioners?

____

____

7) What is this specialty's career path?

____

____

8) Other than ASHP, what specialty associations and local contacts exist?

____

____

9) What recommendations would you make to a new practitioner considering this specialty?

____

____

10) What attributes do you think are important in anyone considering this specialty?

____

____

11) If you had it to do over again would you choose this field of health-system pharmacy? Why or why not?

____

____

12) Who else would you suggest I speak with? May I let them know you referred me?

____

____

Chapter 2

Professional Development

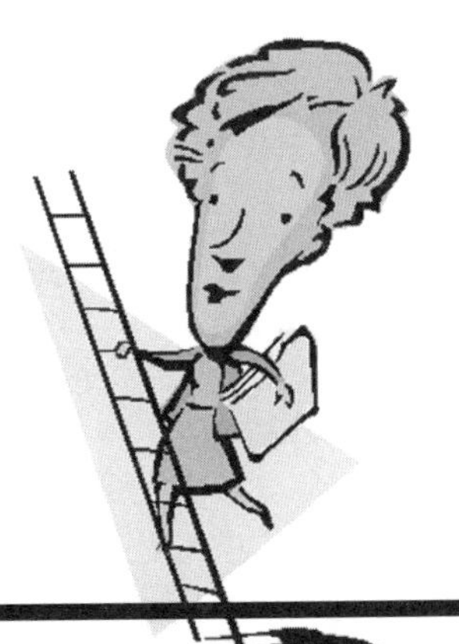

In this chapter we address the topic of professional development—from keeping your curriculum vitae (CV) current to continuing education. If "chance favors the prepared mind," then keeping yourself current will help increase your options and make you ready for whatever might come your way. Specifically, we look at tips for writing a CV, interviewing effectively, networking, and obtaining additional education and certifications.

Curriculum Vitae

The primary purpose of a CV is to get an interview for a potential new job or residency program. A CV is *not* an autobiography. It is *not* an entire work history. It is *not* intended to be the means by which an interviewer decides whether or not to hire you. The CV should provide enough *relevant* information about you so that someone can decide whether or not you should be interviewed.

Many people think a CV and a résumé are the same. Although the two are similar, there are some basic differences. A résumé is rarely longer than a page or two and contains very specific information about your education and experiences. A good CV, on the other hand, is a more in-depth account of your education, achievements, and experiences (e.g., student organization participation, internships, and clinical rotations). A CV should depict your education, experience, and potential for success. It takes time to create an impressive CV. If you don't already have one, you should create one now. If you already have a CV, you should review it carefully and update it every six to twelve months regardless of whether you are planning to apply for a residency, advanced graduate training, or a new job.

If you have never created a CV, you might consider reading *Résumés and Personal Statements for Health Professionals* by James W. Tysinger. You may purchase this book through ASHP by visiting the Web site at www.ashp.org. This book offers a step-by-step approach to starting a CV and offers many samples. Another resource is the article by Kathryn K. Bucci, "How to prepare a curriculum vitae" (*Am J Hosp Pharm.* [1993]; 50:2298–9). In addition, ask current residents or professors for examples of CVs and guidance in preparing yours.

When preparing your CV, describe your experiences in a way that demonstrates that you are an extremely mature, qualified, and responsible individual. Be sure that all information is presented clearly and honestly. Do not fabricate information on your CV. Pharmacy is a small world, and employers can easily find out what is untrue—it may take only one phone call. Be certain that your CV is free from errors, including grammar and spelling mistakes. Make sure preceptor and employer names are spelled correctly and that you know all the degrees following their names. A CV with mistakes in it speaks volumes to an interviewer. Once you have put together a rough draft, have someone review it and critique it for you. (See pages 31–34 for a sample CV.)

When writing about your education and experiences, you must be specific and the information must be relevant to the position for which you hope to be interviewed. For example, in describing your academic coursework, using names such as "Phase VI elective" will mean little to people outside your school. Use short phrases to describe types of rotations, such as "(name of institution) clinical pharmacy rotation" or "(name of community) distributional rotation." You should definitely list month-long rotations, but probably not those that lasted less than two weeks. If you went to ambulatory clinics in a longitudinal fashion (once a week for three months), list these, but be specific about the time invested. Whether you include descriptions of each rotation is up to you. Unless activities during the rotation were unusual (e.g., writing a manuscript, compounding veterinary medications), you may want to leave out detailed descriptions of the rotation.You should provide enough information to be descriptive without overloading the reader. If you received an unusual award, you may want to briefly describe it. This includes merit-based scholarships.

When it comes to any pharmacy-related job experience, detailed information should be included. If you had a job loosely associated with pharmacy (e.g., a business or management-related job in health care), include it if it is pertinent to your skills. If you have publications, make sure they are referenced appropriately. Listing a publication that is in press is fine as long as it is really in press. This means that it has been accepted by a journal and that it will be published. It does not mean that it is sitting on your preceptor's desk waiting to be submitted.

Also pay attention to basic CV presentation, such as format and printing. Most people list items on their CV in reverse chronological order. The reverse chronological CV is written with education and training, experience, publications, honors, and all other information presented with the current or most recent data first, the next most recent data second, and so on. Generally, it is best not to include information that is older than 10–15 years because this information is too dated and you have probably moved beyond the older level of experience. If you have recently graduated, this is not likely to be an issue.

So which comes first, education and training or experience? Decide which is more relevant, impressive, and/or more recent. As a recent graduate or new practitioner, your specialized training and degrees are usually the most significant. However, once you have been working for a while, it may be better to move your experience forward and put your education and training later in the CV.

Use a laser printer to make multiple copies of your CV and list of references on cotton bond paper. This paper can be found at any office supply store. Conservative colors of paper, such as white, cream, and light gray are generally best. Try to avoid folding your CV. Distribute your CV by hand, or mail it in a large envelope (9 × 12) with the other application materials.

An Outline for Preparing a Chronological Curriculum Vitae

Your name should stand out and be quickly visible at the top center of the CV. List a phone number at which you can be easily reached, preferably one with an answering machine or voice mail. An e-mail address is almost more important than a phone number.

Career Summary or Qualifications Summary. This isn't a critical section but it is better than an objective statement that essentially reads "To get a job that will use my skills and abilities and may pay me more than I am making now." If you include this section, it will contain:

- A brief, clearly worded statement of what you do, where you do it, and which of your skills are relevant for the desired position.

- Only those skills supported by fact in the body of the CV.

Education and Training. In reverse chronological order, list specialized training programs, colleges, addresses, degrees, and dates of attendance. Include G.P.A. if outstanding and relevant (if you have been out of school more than three years, it is probably no longer relevant); internships, fellowships, honors, major research, significant courses, and work-study may be listed here or under separate headings.

Experience (full-time, part-time, summer, volunteer, internships). Categorize in reverse chronological order. List dates of employment, name and address of work place, and your job title. Describe your accomplishments and specific tasks rather than responsibilities. Emphasize transferable skills, especially as they relate to the new employer. Begin phrases with action verbs such as organized, planned, led, and advised. Omit personal pronouns. Be positive and concise.

Military Service. Describe in detail if the experience enhances your application.

Affiliations (memberships, certifications). Include membership in professional organizations or fraternities (if you aren't a member, *Join*). Mention offices, titles, special duties, achievements, and awards.

Research and Publications. You may want to include this information under the Education and Training section if you have limited research experience or have been listed in only one or two publications. However, if your research experience is extensive and/or you have been published several times (including being listed as first author), then a separate section is advised.

Additional Skills/Information (computer skills, travel, foreign language proficiency). Describe this information if it is unique or includes required relevant skills or experience.

Extracurricular Activities (only if relevant to work). Describe your activities in the same style as work experience. Include examples of leadership, offices held, program planning involvement, etc.

Sample Curriculum Vitae

David R. Hilton
14901 Woodridge Street
Colesville, MD 21201
(301) 555-5555
DrHilton@pharm.edu

EDUCATION

Doctor of Pharmacy, *University of Silver Spring, School of Pharmacy,* Silver Spring, MD (2000)

Bachelor of Science, Biology; *University of St. Michael's,* Annapolis, MD (1996)

PHARMACEUTICAL EXPERIENCE

H. E. Suddarth Hospital, London, MD, *Pharmacy student technician* (1999–Present)

Precisely filled unit dose prescriptions in the OR pharmacy. Refilled Pyxis machines and starter doses on the intensive care units. Conducted pharmacy quality control inspections for the OR pharmacy to prepare for JCAHO surveys.

Kensington Nursing Home, Hyde Park, MD, *Assistant clinical consultant* (1998–1999)

Accurately processed and dispensed unit dose and multi-dose prescriptions for nursing home and assisted living residents. Surveyed medication administration records for mistakes and discrepancies. Packaged unit dose medications. Performed supervised compounding of topical agents for nursing home inpatients. Delivered medications to nursing home units and assisted living facilities. Made supervised therapy recommendations to nursing home medical staff. Collected clinical data for DUR studies on warfarin and phenytoin monitoring. Assisted with developing lab monitoring sheets for the medical office of an assisted living facility.

CDLA Discount Drugs, Finksburg, MD, *Pharmacy technician* (1997–1998)

Carefully entered and filled prescription orders. Processed refill orders and called for refill approvals from physicians' offices. Answered insurance questions for customers and assisted them in filling out reimbursement forms. Reconstituted oral liquids and topicals for dispensing.

Prescriptotech Pharmaceuticals, Annapolis, MD, *Data entry technician* (1996–1997)

Processed phase III clinical data for a large multi-center study investigating a new drug for heart failure patients. Corrected mistyped drugs and adverse events that were unrecognizable by the statistical database.

David R. Hilton -2-

HONORS & AWARDS

University of Silver Spring

Phi Lambda Sigma leadership honor society (October 1999)
ASHP Student Leadership Award (February 1999)
Rho Chi recognition certificate for scholastic achievement (May 1999)
University of Silver Spring School of Pharmacy leadership award (May 1999)
State of Maryland Senatorial Scholarship for academic achievement (September 1997)

University of St. Michael's

Hughes Undergraduate Biological Science Education grant (September 1993)
Undergraduate Research Opportunity Program grant (September 1994)

PUBLICATIONS, POSTER SESSIONS, AND SENIOR THESIS

Watkins L.R., Wiertelak E.P., Goehler L.E., *Hilton, D.R.*, Martin D., Reile, D.M. Characterization of cytokine-induced hyperalgesia. *Brain Research* 2000; 654(1): 15–26.

Reile, DM, *Hilton, D.R.*, Furness L., Mooney-Heiberger K., Mayr T., Maier S.F., Watkins L.R. Acute and conditioned hyperalgesic responses to illness. *Pain* 1999; 56(2): 227–34.

Watkins L.R., Reile, D.M., Goehler L.E., Mooney Heiberger K., Martinez R., Fumess L., *Hilton, D.R.*, Maier S.F. Neurocircuitry of illness-induced hyperalgesia. *Brain Research* 1998; 639(2): 283–99.

Watkins L.R., Reile, D.M., Furness L., *Hilton, D.R.*, Martinez R., Maier S.F. Neurocircuitry of centrifugal pain facilitory systems: anti-analgesia and hyperalgesia. Poster presentation. Society for Neuroscience annual meeting 1997.

LPS-induced hyperalgesia measured by both the tail-flick and formalin tests of pain sensitivity. Senior Thesis. University of St. Michael's, Department of Behavioral Neuropsychology, 1996.

RESEARCH EXPERIENCE

University of St. Michael's, Department of Behavioral Neuropsychology Laboratory (1995–1996)

Assisted with development of a rodent model for illness-induced hyperalgesia. Performed rodent spinal cord and brain dissection and other histology techniques for neurocircuitry studies. Conducted rodent conditioning sessions for studies of antianalgesia and conditioned analgesia. Assisted with rodent stereotaxic surgeries and performed post-op care duties. Trained other undergraduate students in rat handling and conditioning techniques.

Supervisor: David M. Reile, Ph.D.

David R. Hilton -3-

Kensington Nursing Home, Hyde Park, MD (1998–1999)

Collected clinical data for a research study on anticoagulation strategies and warfarin monitoring in five different nursing home facilities. Results were presented in a poster session at the American Society of Consultant Pharmacists annual meeting, November 1998.

Supervisor: B. Hilton, R.Ph.

EXTRACURRICULAR ACTIVITIES

American Society of Health-System Pharmacists, University of Silver Spring School of Pharmacy, student society founding member and president (1998–1999)

American Society of Health-System Pharmacists, University of Silver Spring School of Pharmacy, student liaison (1998–1999)

Alpha Zeta Omega pharmacy fraternity member (1997–current)

PRESENTATIONS

New treatment options for Parkinson's disease, Geriatric clinic in-service

Veterans Administration Medical Center, Baltimore, Maryland (1999)

Idiopathic thrombocytopenic purpura, Pharmacy staff in-service

University of Silver Spring Hospital (1998)

Pathophysiology and treatment of sickle cell disease in adolescent patients, Pharmacy staff in-service, Howard University Hospital (1998)

EXPERIENTIAL ROTATIONS

Institutional Pharmacy: Inpatient pharmacy, State of Maryland Psychiatric Hospital, Sykesville, MD; July–August 1997, Janice Keys, R.Ph

Community Pharmacy: Seek's Pharmacy, Four Corners, MD; August–September 1997, Dwight C. Seek, R.Ph.

Community Clinical Pharmacy: CDLA Discount Drug, Finksburg, MD; September–October 1997, JoAnn Harris, R.Ph.

Institutional Clinical Pharmacy: Pediatric pharmacy, University of Silver Spring Hospital, Silver Spring, MD; October–November 1997, Doris A. Smith, R.Ph.

Outpatient Clinic: Anticoagulation clinic, Catholic University Hospital, Washington, DC; January–February 1998, Pat A. McWilliams, R.Ph.

David R. Hilton -4-

Outpatient Clinic: Geriatric clinic, VA Medical Center, Baltimore, MD; March–April 1998, Jonathan Pestle, R.Ph.

Elective Pharmacy Experience: Investigational drug service, Maryland Research Hospital, Baltimore, MD; May–June 1999, D. R. Michaels, R.Ph.

Elective Pharmacy Experience: Montgomery County Poison Control Center, Rockville, MD; July–August 1999, Deborah Thurlow, R.Ph.

Elective Pharmacy Experience: Drug Information Service, Silver Spring University Hospital, Silver Spring, MD; October–November 1999, Angela C. Stevens, R.Ph.

PROFESSIONAL ORGANIZATIONS

American Society of Health-System Pharmacists
Maryland Society of Health-System Pharmacists
American Pharmaceutical Association—Academy of Students of Pharmacy
University of St. Michael's Pharmaceutical Association

REFERENCES

William Phileas, Pharm.D.
Allied Health Building
100 Georgia Avenue
Silver Spring, MD 20910
(301) 555-3274

Roberta Bernhardt, Pharm.D., BCPS
Allied Health Building
100 Georgia Avenue
Silver Spring, MD 20910
(301) 555-3278

George Reagan, R.Ph.
Pharmaceutical Services
6105 Washington Road
Colesville, MD 20852
(301) 555-2987

Interviewing

The purpose of an interview (whether for a job, a residency, or a fellowship) is to determine the suitability between you and the organization. This process focuses on three areas:

- Credentials—Do you have the necessary skills and experience to do the work?
- Initiative—Are you a self-starter or do you need constant monitoring?
- Match—What kind of person are you? Will you fit in with the existing staff?

When evaluating these questions, it is important to remember that interviewing is a mutual process. In other words, while you are being evaluated by the organization, you are also evaluating the position to see if it is a good fit and a sound choice for you at this point in your career. "How to be interviewed for a job" by G.R. Hasegawa (*Am J Hosp Pharm.* [1991]; 48:1180 and1183) contains additional general interviewing advice.

Types and Formats of Interviews. There are a variety of types and formats for interviews. These vary depending on the position (job or residency) and organization (hospital, university, clinic, etc.). Most interviews will fit into one of two types: initial and hiring.

Initial or *screening interviews* are designed to reduce the number of applicants for a position to a few top candidates. The typical format is a one-on-one, face-to-face interview although the group interview is not uncommon. It may be as short as 20 minutes to an hour or as long as a full morning or afternoon for higher-level positions. The average residency or fellowship interview is about six hours.

Hiring interviews take place after applicants have passed the initial interview stage. Hiring interviews may be significantly more in-depth, in terms of both time and job-related content. They often involve more than one interviewer and you are likely to be presented with questions about salary and benefits. However, if the initial interview was lengthy, selection may come in the form of an offer letter or a phone call rather than a face-to-face meeting.

Formats for interviews vary and include not only the typical individual interview but also telephone interviews, serial interviews, and group interviews. If you expect to receive a phone interview, keep your application materials and CV near the phone. This will help you to refer to information quickly during the interview. Serial interviews involve meeting individually with several different interviewers. The key here is to pace yourself. It is understandable that you will get tired and frustrated with answering the same questions over and over. However it is not uncommon for the director or another senior person to be the final interviewer, so you need to appear fresh and interested (even when you don't feel that way).

Finally, group interviews can take at least two forms. In the first format, you are interviewed by several interviewers at the same time. In the second, you are interviewed with several other applicants at the same time. If you are interviewed by a group, make sure that you make eye contact with each person during the interview and pay attention to the group dynamics. If you are interested in a residency or fellowship program that accepts several residents, there will probably be other applicants interviewing with you on the same day. Some activities, such as lunch, the tour, and information sessions will be shared with other applicants. During the actual interviewing, you may be alone with one or more interviewers. If you are interviewed with a group of other applicants, make sure that you interact with the interviewers. You don't have to be aggressive and take control of the interview, but you must not shrink back and be quiet. You may not like the other applicants but try not to let it show. It is quite possible that you will be working with some or all of these people next year. Part of the residency involves working as a team; so you need to portray that you can work well with others, even if you are in competition.

Interview Preparation. One key to successful interviewing is preparation. When you receive a call inviting you for an interview, ask what the interview will be like (format, length, etc.). This way, you will know what to expect. Knowing the title or role of the interviewer might also provide some clue as to the tone and formality level to expect.

Here are some fundamental areas that may guide you in your preparation:

- *Personal background.* Read and re-read your CV so you can talk comfortably about your experience, education, and training without looking at your notes.

- *Needed materials.* Find out in advance what materials you will need to bring to the interview. In addition to extra copies of your CV, you may need transcripts; training certificates; letters of reference or names, addresses, and phone numbers of references; and writing samples.

Clinical Specialists

Rita K. Jew, Pharm.D.

Pharmacy Clinical Coordinator & Clinical Specialist in Neonatology, The Children's Hospital of Philadelphia

Dr. Rita Jew began practicing in 1991. After earning a Pharm.D. degree from the University of California–San Francisco School of Pharmacy, she completed an ASHP-accredited residency in clinical pharmacy at Thomas Jefferson University Hospital in Philadelphia, Pennsylvania. She also completed the ASHP Competitive Edge Program, advanced experimental training in conducting and using outcome studies. Before accepting the Clinical Coordinator position at Children's Hospital of Philadelphia, Dr. Jew worked as a clinical pharmacist.

Dr. Jew has numerous responsibilities. As clinical coordinator, she establishes and expands clinical pharmacy services. She supervises six clinicians and coordinates all clinical and administrative activities in her department. She develops goals and service initiatives for comprehensive pharmaceutical care services, participates in institutional and departmental committees, including Continuous Quality Improvement initiatives and the therapeutic standards committee. Dr. Jew edits the pharmacy newsletter, edits and reviews the hospital formulary, and maintains the hospital formulary system. She is active in program development and coordinates programs in drug-use evaluation, adverse-reaction reporting, investigational drugs, staff development, a mini-residency program for staff pharmacists, pharmacology and pharmacokinetics consultative services for other health care professionals, and a pharmacy-based intervention program. Additionally, Dr. Jew provides pharmaceutical care services to the neonatal intensive care team.

Dr. Jew has been active in professional organizations and states, "These activities have given me a much broader sense of what the issues are in the pharmacy community. It has given me excellent networking opportunities and exposed me to areas and people in pharmacy that I would otherwise not be exposed to. My exposure has definitely helped in resolving issues at my job." Perhaps this is one reason why Dr. Jew takes such an active educational approach on the job. She provides inservices, lectures, and grand rounds for medical, pharmacy, and nursing staff. Dr. Jew is a preceptor for the pediatric pharmacy practice residency and the clinical clerkship program for Doctor of Pharmacy candidates.

Dr. Jew's involvement with ASHP on the national level includes serving

continued next page

Rita K. Jew, Pharm.D. *(continued)*

as the Director-at-Large on the Section of Clinical Specialists' Executive Committee and as a mentor with the ASHP Practice Advancement Links Program. She has also been involved professionally on the state and local levels, as a member of the Pennsylvania Society of Health-System Pharmacists' Task Force for Student Section and the Council of Organizational Affairs and as member and chair of the membership committee. She has also served the Delaware Valley Society of Health-System Pharmacists as president-elect, chair of the nominations committee, member of the Board of Directors, and chair of the membership committee. It should come as no surprise then that Dr. Jew recommends making professional involvement a part of your career. She states, "Do it while you are not too preoccupied with other things in life. However, know your limits, and do not over-commit."

From the hiring standpoint, Dr. Jew acknowledges that since the Pharm.D. is now an entry-level degree, she looks for someone with residency training. When looking to fill her clinical specialist positions, she expects someone with a pharmacy practice residency and a second year of pediatric specialty training. Finally, Dr. Jew offers these words to new practitioners, "Dedication and enthusiasm in your pharmacy career is what makes you a good practitioner. Caring about your patients is what makes you a great practitioner. Remember, your primary focus is your patients!"

- *Organizational and field knowledge.* Be familiar with major developments and trends in pharmacy and in your field of interest, as well as the mission and direction of the organization interviewing you.

- *Logistical preparation.* Know in advance where you are going and how to get there. Make certain that you have detailed directions, especially if you are going to a city you've never been to before. Allow plenty of time to get to the interview. There is nothing more stressful to an applicant than missing a bus, trying to find parking, or getting lost on the way to an interview.

- *Clothing and appearance.* Many qualified applicants have lost job offers because of poor grooming or inappropriate clothing. Dress to fit the organization; tend toward the conservative. It is probably always better to dress up than to dress too casually. Jewelry and make-up should complement, not distract from, the overall look. Facial hair on men should be neat and trimmed. You want to be remembered for your professionalism and ability, not what you look like. Cologne or perfume should be applied moderately as some people are allergic and may react negatively to certain scents.

Interview Components. Most interviews have elements in common: the introduction, the interview questions themselves, and the closing. Each is important for different reasons, and your success depends on knowing how to respond appropriately in each segment.

- *The introduction.* You may have heard all you need to know about a firm handshake and making eye contact. What you may not have heard is that many hiring decisions are made within the first 30–45 seconds. This points not only to the importance of appearance and proper grooming but also to your social and interpersonal skills. Remember, it is expected that, if offered the position, you can and will do the job. The interview is a time to confirm that and also to determine whether or not you will "fit in" with the organization. First impressions influence interviewers' decisions.

- *Interview questions.* Most of your preparation for the interview should focus on performing well at this stage. Even though some of the interview process is subjective and focuses on fit, interviewers are still primarily looking for individuals who can do the work. During this stage of the interview, you have the opportunity to offer an honest appraisal of your strengths and skills and to show why you are well suited for the position. The next section provides questions you can review to help in your preparation.

As previously stated, the average residency or fellowship interview lasts about six hours. Job interviews tend to be significantly shorter, although not always. If the interview is scheduled to last all day or over the lunch hour, you will probably eat with members of the staff at some point either at a restaurant or in the cafeteria. Occasionally, residency directors or others may offer to take you out to dinner or you may be asked to go to happy hour with the preceptors, residents, other applicants, and staff. Whether you decide to have an alcoholic drink is entirely up to you, with a few exceptions. Do not order an alcoholic drink at lunch; do not consume more than two drinks under any circumstances; and do not feel compelled to order an alcoholic drink if everybody else does.

When applying for a residency, you will want to speak with the current residents if you can get them away from the faculty or preceptors. They will provide the most insightful information about the residency. It is very important that you ask them whether they would choose this residency again, if given the chance. If they say no, be sure to ask them why. The reasons they give for not liking the program may be something that is irrelevant to your situation.

- *The close.* As the interview draws toward a close, you may need to offer a summary of your strengths in response to such questions as "Why should we offer the position to you?" You will also need to show interest and enthusiasm for the position and end the interview with another firm handshake and good eye contact. Additionally, you may be asked if you have any questions for the interviewer(s). No matter what, you must not respond with "No." If all of your questions have been answered, ask if you can have a brief tour of the facility or if you can meet some of the people with whom you will be working. It is appropriate to state that all of your major questions have been answered, but that you would like to emphasize your strong interest in the position. At least this response gives you another chance to "sell yourself."

Interview Questions. During your various interviews, you will be asked many questions. It is important that you mentally prepare answers to some of the most common. It is unlikely that you will get many questions as hard as some of the ones listed below. The following is a random sampling to let you know what you might come across. Make sure that you know your CV backwards and forwards! Any question they ask you about is fair game. If you have done an inservice on a pharmacy-related topic and it is mentioned on your CV, review your notes or handouts prior to interviews since it is possible they may ask you something about it.

It is also extremely important that you be prepared to ask plenty of questions. Interviewers often make judgments about you based on the type of questions you ask. Some questions should be directed to residents, if at all. Do not attempt to ask all of these questions. Ask the most crucial questions in the limited amount of time you may be given.

Common Interview Questions. As tempting as it might be to memorize sample responses from interview books, avoid this trap. Savvy interviewers will see through "canned" answers, and you may come off looking overly slick or contrived. Answers should sound well thought-out, but not memorized.

Interview questions typically come from such topic areas as education, training, personal traits, pharmacy experience, and career goals. In a new trend, called behavioral interviewing, applicants might also be asked to discuss how they would handle a specific work-related situation.

Practitioner Spotlight

Clinical Specialists

Marianne Billeter, Pharm.D., BCPS

Associate Professor of Pharmacy Practice
Coordinator, Nontraditional Practice Curriculum, Division of Distance Education, Bernard J. Dunn School of Pharmacy, Shenandoah University

Dr. Marianne Billeter has been with Shenandoah University for four years. She started at Shenandoah when the second pharmacy class was entering and has been part of the unique building process of starting a new college of pharmacy. Shenandoah graduated its first pharmacy class in May of 2000.

Dr. Billeter's primary responsibility is teaching. She teaches courses in infectious diseases, health promotion and disease prevention, and contemporary issues in pharmacy practice. She also does a number of guest lectures in a variety of other courses within the School of Pharmacy, usually related to infectious diseases or HIV/AIDS. Outside of pharmacy, she lectures on basic immunology, antibiotic management, and HIV/AIDS in the Division of Nursing at the master's degree level. Although she currently does not have an active clinical practice, she works closely with the infection control department at the Winchester Medical Center.

Dr. Billeter's other responsibilities are in the Division of Distance Education. The school offers a Pharm.D. degree to practicing pharmacists, using a nontraditional, distance education model over the Internet. She helps to answer questions for more than one hundred seventy active students. She is responsible for the creation of the exams students take throughout the program and for facilitating the experiential component of the degree.

In addition to Dr. Billeter's teaching and administrative responsibilities, she is the faculty advisor for the Alpha Chi Chapter of Kappa Epsilon Fraternity and was the advisor for the student affiliate chapter of the Virginia Society of Health-System Pharmacists. She states, "The student leadership in this group has been a real pleasure to work with . . . . They are refocusing the organization and, in the process, jump-starting it to gain more membership."

Dr. Billeter received a bachelor of science in pharmacy and a Pharm.D. from Purdue University. During her clinical rotations, she became interested in infectious diseases and HIV/AIDS. She went on to complete a two-year residency in clinical pharmacy at the A.B. Chandler Medical Center at the University of Kentucky. During her residency, her interest in infectious diseases strengthened and she continued her training with a fellowship in infectious diseases at the University of Kentucky.

continued next page

Marianne Billeter, Pharm.D., BCPS *(continued)*

Dr. Billeter obtained her first job at Xavier University College of Pharmacy and remained there for seven years. At Xavier, she taught infectious diseases in the therapeutics course and had an active clinical practice at the Ochsner Medical Institutions, where she went on rounds with the physicians on the infectious disease service. During her time at Xavier, Dr. Billeter gave presentations, published articles, developed a national reputation, and was granted tenure.

She credits ASHP and the Louisiana Society of Health-System Pharmacists (LSHP) with helping in the development of her professional career. She praises the accredited residency training opportunities and Personnel Placement Service ASHP offers new practitioners. During her fellowship, Dr. Billeter became a part of ASHP's Infectious Disease Specialty Practice Group, eventually becoming vice chair. Since ASHP developed the Section of Clinical Specialists, Dr. Billeter has been involved in this section, serving on various committees, and now as a member of the Executive Committee of the Section of Clinical Specialists. Dr. Billeter also served on the Commission on Therapeutics for three years. Through her involvement in the LSHP, Dr. Billeter began speaking at various local meetings, then at larger conventions, and eventually was invited to speak at the ASHP Midyear Clinical Meeting. Dr. Billeter states, "With all of this, I can truly say that ASHP and LSHP have helped to develop and refine my career as a clinical pharmacist."

Dr. Billeter advises new practitioners to become involved. She says, "Don't let your profession just pass you by; get involved and help shape your profession." In interviewing for hiring purposes, she stresses the importance of good communication skills.

Questions most frequently asked in a variety of job interviews and settings include the following:

1. Tell me about yourself.
2. What are your strengths and weaknesses?
3. Why are you leaving your current position? Why did you leave your last job? (If relevant to your situation.)
4. What attracts you to this organization/setting/position?
5. Where do you see yourself in five to ten years?

6. What do you think makes you best qualified for the position?
7. What do you think you can contribute to this position/organization/department/staff?
8. What is the salary you are looking for in this position? (If relevant to your situation.)
9. Tell me about a project that you handled well and one in which you were not successful. What did you learn from each one?
10. Do you have any questions?

Questions asked in a pharmacy setting might include the following:

1. What do you want to get out of a residency?
2. Why do you want to come here?
3. Describe a clinical intervention you have made.
4. What practice areas are you interested in?
5. How much hospital experience have you had?
6. What is one of the major issues facing pharmacy today?
7. What would your pharmacy preceptors say about you?
8. What would your colleagues say about you?
9. Would relocating be a problem?
10. What were your least favorite rotations and why?
11. What qualities do you expect in a preceptor?
12. Do you have any ideas for your major project?
13. How do you handle stress?
14. Have you ever had a major conflict with a preceptor/doctor? If so, how did you handle it?

Thought or reaction questions and behavioral interviewing questions might be similar to the following:

1. Here's a scenario we would like you to consider: You are the only pharmacist in the pharmacy. On the phone is a nurse wanting to know dosing for a dopamine drip for a patient who is crashing. At the window is a doctor who is ranting and raving about an enoxaparin order that wasn't approved. On the other line is a nurse calling about a patient with a vancomycin level of 15. In what order do you handle these problems?

2. How would you deal with an unmotivated student?

3. If you were alone on a deserted island, what three medications would you bring with you?

4. What makes you better for this position than other candidates?

5. What do you anticipate a typical day in your career to be like?

6. If you could be any drug, what drug would you be and why?

7. Choose a topic relating to clinical pharmacy, and we'll ask you a question about it.

Potentially Difficult Questions. Every interview candidate dreads being asked certain questions. No matter how much you prepare and practice, you are likely to be asked one or two questions that leave you searching for the right response. Potentially difficult topic areas might include breaks between employment, getting low marks in a class or a rotation, having been fired or laid off, and the like. In addition, you may be asked illegal or inappropriate questions about your personal life (e.g., questions about your family life or marital status). Anticipate and prepare for the very questions you are most concerned about answering. Here are some other guidelines to include:

- *Think before answering.* There is nothing wrong with pausing a few moments before responding to a tough question. Say something like, "That's a good question. I'd like to take a moment to think before I respond." This gives you a chance to collect your thoughts and may result in the interviewer pulling back on an illegal or inappropriate question.

Acute Care

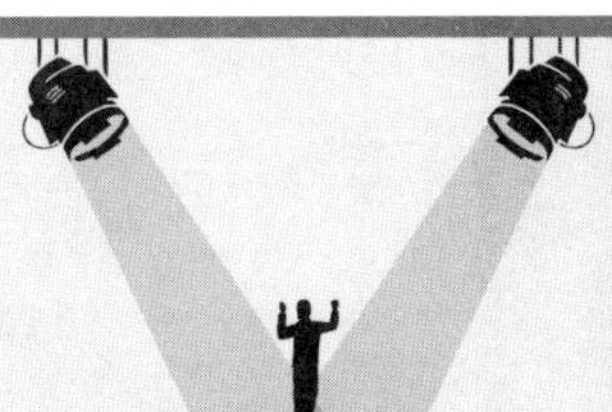

Burnis D. Breland, Pharm.D., M.S.

Director of Pharmacy and Clinical Research, Columbus Regional Healthcare System
Adjunct Associate Professor of Clinical Pharmacy Practice, Auburn University
Preceptor, University of Georgia and Mercer University Schools of Pharmacy

Practitioner Spotlight

As the Director of Pharmacy—a position he has held for the past sixteen years—Dr. Burnis Breland's day involves planning, organizing, staffing, and monitoring all departmental operations. Such work includes personnel and financial management, development and maintenance of clinical programs, and oversight of the purchasing of and contracting for pharmaceuticals. As the Director of Clinical Research for the past five years, Dr. Breland also oversees the activities of the clinical research specialists who coordinate various research protocols.

Dr. Breland started in the world of pharmacy by practicing as a intern in a community pharmacy before graduation. After receiving a B.S. degree in pharmacy, he completed an ASHP-accredited residency in hospital pharmacy. He obtained additional experience by working part-time as a staff pharmacist in various hospitals and in a community pharmacy while awaiting entrance into graduate school. Dr. Breland obtained a master of science degree in hospital pharmacy and then served as a supervisor of the Intravenous Admixture and Hyperalimentation program at Hermann Hospital in Houston, Texas. This administrative frontline job provided him with valuable experience in practicing and managing at a large institution.

Dr. Breland returned to school and completed a Pharm.D. degree, after which he became Assistant Professor of Clinical Pharmacy Practice at the University of Mississippi. For the next several years, Dr. Breland taught and worked as a clinical practitioner at various institutions. After founding the Department of Clinical Research at Columbus Regional five years ago, Dr. Breland has served as the department's director.

Throughout his education, training, and employment, Dr. Breland has been an intern, resident, staff pharmacist, supervisory pharmacist, associate director, and director. The experience he obtained in working at different hospitals and health systems, as well as in community pharmacy, has provided him with the knowledge and experience needed to develop pharmacy

continued next page

Burnis D. Breland, Pharm.D., M.S. *(continued)*

programs within an integrated health care system, including ambulatory, home care, long-term care, acute care, and managed care.

Dr. Breland has been a member of ASHP since his senior year in pharmacy school in 1974. He has been an active member of ASHP and various local and state pharmacy organizations. With ASHP, he has been chairman of the Council on Professional Affairs and the Practice Management Group and is a current member of the Council on Administrative Affairs. He emphasizes, "ASHP has proven to be an excellent source of continuing education and collaboration with other practitioners."

Dr. Breland stresses that new practitioners must strive to obtain the best education and training experiences available to them. Obtaining a Pharm.D. degree is now essential, and he highly recommends completing a pharmacy practice residency, followed by a specialty residency. He recommends that new practitioners look for a mentor and become active with local and state pharmacy organizations.

Dr. Breland concludes by saying, "Pharmacy practice in the acute care setting is dynamic and challenging, but can be both professionally and personally rewarding." Practicing pharmacy in the acute care setting provides an excellent opportunity for pharmacists to use their extensive knowledge of pharmacology and therapeutics and to have a significant impact on the health outcome of patients. The broad scope of practice in the acute care setting of today's health systems provides the opportunity for practitioners to practice in one area, obtain expertise, and then move to other areas if their interests change. Pharmacists practicing in the acute care setting work with and learn from other health care professionals and work as a team member in the provision of care to patients.

- *Ask the interviewer to restate the question.* If you don't understand what is being asked, ask the interviewer to restate the question. Often, this simple request can alert the interviewer to the fact that he or she has asked the question poorly—or perhaps, in an illegal way. The restated question is likely to be clearer and less difficult to answer.

- *Be brief and respond in a factual way.* Interviewees often volunteer more information than is necessary. For example, when asked why you left a previous position, you should avoid saying anything negative about a supervisor (even if it is true). Instead, focus on the skills you hope to bring from a previous position into the new one.

- *Focus on what is really being asked.* Questions about age, marriage, and family care issues can sometimes be addressed positively by going to the heart of the interviewer's concern. For instance, a woman does not have to answer whether or not she has children; but if this seems to be an issue for the interviewer, she might consider responding, "My career is very important to me and will continue to be and I can assure you that I am dedicated to quality care as a pharmacist."

- *Never lie, exaggerate, or overstate.* When asked direct questions about your work, experience, training, or ability to handle key elements of the job, you must respond honestly. Many organizations will fire individuals immediately if they are found to have lied in an interview. Not only is honesty the best policy; in most cases, deception will only cause more problems for you later on.

Asking Questions. It is important to plan questions to ask during the interview. Remember that this is a time for you to evaluate the organization, residency, or fellowship. Following is a list of questions you might consider asking in a residency interview and those you might reserve for current residents only. You may also adapt questions from these lists if you are interviewing for a new pharmacy position.

Questions to Ask in General

1. Is code team participation required or optional?
2. How many hours are spent with service commitments per week/month?
3. Are residents ever pulled from clinical areas for service commitments?
4. Can rotations be changed during the year?
5. How easy is it to get a desired elective rotation?
6. How is the topic of the residency project decided?
7. Are there any opportunities to teach or precept pharmacy students?
8. Are there any opportunities to publish?
9. Is it possible to do a rotation at another institution?

10. How do you think this year's residents are doing?

11. What are the current residents' research projects?

12. What are the strengths and weaknesses of the program?

13. What will participation in the program do for me?

14. How are residents evaluated during the program?

15. Do the pharmacy faculty ever work with the medical faculty on research projects?

16. How would you describe the relationship between the distributional pharmacists and the clinical pharmacists or residents?

17. Are residents given the opportunity to attend national pharmacy meetings (e.g., ASHP, APhA, ACCP, SCCM)? If so, is funding available?

18. Do pharmacists or residents ever give lectures to medical house staff?

19. Can residents select their own ambulatory clinic?

20. What clinics are available?

21. Is it possible to tailor the structure of the residency to meet my interests (infectious disease, pediatrics, etc.)?

Questions to Consider Asking Only Residents (or other staff)

1. What is your typical day like?

2. What time do you get to work, on average?

3. Have you had any problems working with the residency director/preceptor?

4. Do you ever spend time with the other residents outside of work?

5. What do you plan to do next year?

6. What would you change about this residency program?

7. What are the best and worst things about this residency?

Acute Care

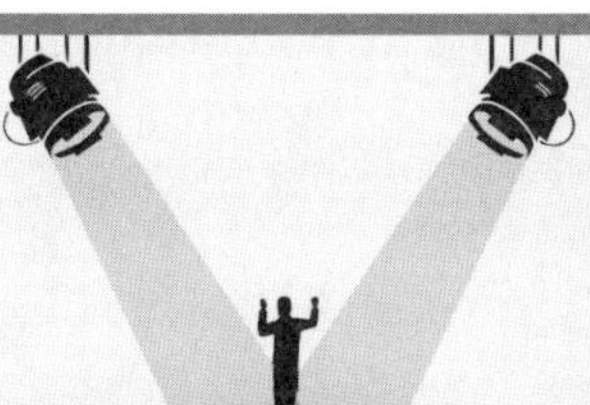

Keith M. Olsen, Pharm.D., FCCP

Associate Professor of Pharmacy, University of Nebraska Medical Center
Critical Care Clinical Specialist, Nebraska Health System

Dr. Keith Olsen's fifteen years of experience include work as an educator and as a clinical specialist in adult intensive care. As an educator, he is a preceptor for pharmacy students and residents doing their critical care rotation, participating in rounds with the critical care medicine team. Occasionally, he assists the pharmacy in staff development and serves on hospital committees. Dr. Olsen lectures in therapeutics and conducts research related to patients in the critical care unit. During Dr. Olsen's critical care career he has worked closely with medical, surgical, intensive care, and nutrition support teams and has created and directed a pharmacokinetic consulting service for a university hospital. Dr. Olsen is a prolific writer who has authored over 150 works.

Dr. Olsen is a member of the ASHP Commission on Therapeutics. He assisted in the development of therapeutic guidelines on stress ulcer prophylaxis, served as critical care facilitator for the Clinical Specialists Section, and published articles in *AJHP* and *Clinical Pharmacy*. Dr. Olsen states, "Like any society activity, interaction with other practitioners is the greatest reward for an individual. My observations of other people, sharing of ideas and experiences, and professional networking have been invaluable to me."

Dr. Olsen's recommendation for new practitioners is to become involved with an organization and an institution. He urges new practitioners to document their activities and to develop programs that alter the outcomes of the patients they treat. He strongly encourages new practitioners to attend national meetings to network and to hear cutting edge continuing-education presentations. Finally, Dr. Olsen exhorts practitioners, "Use your eagerness and energy to tap older practitioners' knowledge to improve your skills; [hold on to them] and learn what you can from these people. [And] always remember, the more you work and read, the more you find out what you don't know. Use that understanding to motivate yourself to be the best practitioner you can."

8. Is photocopying paid for or is there an allowance?
9. How accessible is the library?
10. Are you ever on call?
11. What do you do on the weekends?
12. Do you have to pay for parking?
13. Are the medical and nursing staff easy to work with at this institution?
14. Are health, life, dental, and disability insurance and retirement benefits provided or available?
15. How many calls have you received in the middle of the night while on call?
16. Do the current residents work well together?
17. How far do you live from work?
18. How long does it take you to get to work?
19. Is the neighborhood near the institution safe?
20. Have you had the opportunity to give lectures to pharmacy students? How many?
21. Have you received enough positive or negative feedback throughout your residency?
22. What is the policy for working on holidays?
23. Have you had the opportunity to write or publish during the residency (review articles, hospital newsletter articles, case reports)?
24. Do you have free time after work? How do you spend your free time?
25. Are your suggestions to medical staff taken seriously?
26. How much impact do you have on drug therapy decisions?
27. Are you asked for input?

Presentations. Although it is unusual for a pharmacy practice residency (not for a specialty) to require presentations during an interview, a few programs have asked applicants to give a presentation. Before you decide on a topic or format, ask the program director what is expected in the presentation. Find out what type of topic is preferred, whether audio visual equipment is required and if it will be provided, who your audience will be, and the desired length of your presentation.

Interview Follow-Up. After your interview, be sure to write a formal and succinct thank you note. Writing thank you notes for the residents is a nice touch. You should mail the notes as soon as possible and (if applicable) before the deadline for submitting match results. Letters and envelopes should be addressed with care so that interviewers' names, titles, and degrees are correctly spelled. You should print your letters on good quality paper, using a standard business style.

In addition to writing thank you letters, you should debrief after the interviews. Explore your thoughts about the position—its pros and cons—and any unanswered questions. Think about what you did well in the interview and what areas need further work. This focused debriefing can assist you in continuing to refine your interview skills over time and in learning to think critically about your job search in general.

Networking

Successful career planning doesn't stop once you are accepted into a good residency program or are hired for a great new job. Success within an organization and in your career depends on staying up-to-date on the latest information, techniques, procedures, and medications within health-system pharmacy and staying connected with people. Networking is the ongoing process of building and maintaining relationships with people in your profession.

To many, networking conjures up the image of a smooth talking used car salesman or a desperate job seeker running around professional meetings shaking hands, passing out business cards, and begging others for work. Neither image is a true representation of networking. The most productive networker is one who is friendly and interested in his or her profession; attends local and national meetings; stays active in continuing education; volunteers on different committees; looks for opportunities to teach, write, and do research; and, most importantly, stays involved in a variety of professional activities.

Networking is not complicated or difficult—it simply takes time. It is, however, time well spent. If you look over the profiles in this book you will notice that all practitioners mention their connections with different associations, teaching responsibilities, committee appointments, or research and writing activities. Even new practitioners can get involved just by asking. Check with your local association administrators, and inquire about how you can become more involved. If your preceptor or director asks for volunteers on a research or writing project—volunteer. Read journals and other professional literature to see who's doing what. If you find a topic of interest, be bold and write or e-mail the authors and ask if you can get involved in a project with them. Whenever you connect with a new person or receive help from a colleague, write a thank-you note. It can be brief; in fact, for someone at a peer level a quick e-mail is appropriate. A colleague who is more senior should receive a handwritten note. Above all, stay involved.

Additional Education

Post-Baccalaureate Doctor of Pharmacy Degree. In 1992 a majority of schools and colleges of pharmacy in the United States voted to move toward awarding the Pharm.D. degree as the only professional degree in pharmacy. Currently, only two pharmacy colleges and schools offer the B.S. of pharmacy degree to new students. Starting in fall 2002, all new pharmacy students will enter a Pharm.D. program.

In order to qualify to take the licensure examination in all states, students must graduate from an accredited pharmacy program. A Pharm.D. program is designed as a comprehensive professional curriculum and requires at least four academic years of professional study and a minimum of two years of pre-professional (undergraduate) study, for a total of six to eight years of study after high school. Individual schools have specific requirements for pre-professional study.

As the transition to the Pharm.D. degree continues, many schools and colleges of pharmacy have developed programs to assist practitioners in acquiring the skills and knowledge they need to continue to be successful and competitive. These nontraditional educational programs are offered to practitioner students at a number of schools and are designed as post-baccalaureate degrees, with a combined period of study usually exceeding six years. These programs provide education through a variety of instructional methods including distance learning techniques, such as videotaped lectures, interactive computer, or satellite television. For additional information, go to the Web site of the American Association of Colleges of Pharmacy (http://www.aacp.org/Students/pharmacyeducation.html).

Other Degrees (M.B.A., MPH, M.S., Ph.D.). Another increasingly common career path for students and new practitioners is the completion of advanced graduate study. Advanced degree programs in one of the pharmaceutical sciences may lead to a master of science (M.S.) or doctor of philosophy (Ph.D.) degree. These require an undergraduate degree at least at the bachelor's level prior to enrollment; however, the undergraduate degree need not be in pharmacy. The M.S. and Ph.D. degrees are research degrees and do not qualify the student to be a licensed pharmacy practitioner, unless the student has also earned a B.S. in pharmacy or Pharm.D. degree. Some opt to study outside of pharmacy and earn a juris doctor (J.D.) degree in law or a master of business administration (M.B.A.) degree. Depending on your career path, especially in research facilities or as a professor, you may choose to pursue an advanced graduate degree.

Board Certification

After completing a Pharm.D. degree (whether traditionally or nontraditionally), there are a number of credentialing opportunities. This first step is passing your state's licensing exam. You become a registered pharmacist upon successful completion of your state's licensing exam and are allowed to legally practice pharmacy in a particular state.

Other credentialing opportunities include certificate training programs, traineeships, residencies, and fellowships. Additionally, a pharmacist who wishes to may achieve an advanced certification in one or more of ten pharmacy specializations. The Board of Pharmaceutical Specialties administers examinations in and grants the title "board certified" to pharmacists in the areas of nuclear pharmacy, nutrition support pharmacy, oncology pharmacy, pharmacotherapy, and psychiatric pharmacy. The Commission for Certification in Geriatric Pharmacy (CCGP) offers a certificate program for pharmacists who specialize in treating elderly patients. After passing the CCGP exam, a pharmacist earns the Geriatric Certified Pharmacist credential. Additionally, the National Association of Boards of Pharmacy (NABP) administers tests to pharmacists who want to be certified in the management of a specific disease. Pharmacists who pass NABP's test receive certification from the National Institute for Standards in Pharmacist Credentialing. Disease management certification is available in four specialty areas: anticoagulation therapy, asthma, diabetes, and dyslipidemia.

For more information on credentialing, contact the Board of Pharmaceutical Specialties, the Commission for Certification in Geriatric Pharmacy, the National Association of Boards of Pharmacy, or read "Credentialing in Pharmacy" in the *American Journal of Health-System Pharmacy* (2001; 58: 69–76).

Chapter 3

Work Survival Tips

Reality vs. School

School is stressful for many students. Their time and their lives never seem to be their own. There are classes to attend, papers to write, exams to take, rotations to complete, and money may be tight. In school, however, classmates and faculty provide a support system and you have the chance to be idealistic. The opportunities within pharmacy seem limitless.

Once you graduate, you may feel overwhelmed by the possibilities and opportunities facing you. In the workforce, you will find that a shortage of pharmacists is driving salaries up and hospitals and retail pharmacies are competing for new graduates. A recent article in USA*Today* (Pharmacists now can write their own tickets, March 15, 2001, 3B) reported starting salaries for new graduates ranged from $67,000 to $75,000. Some employers offer signing bonuses and expensive cars. If you choose to further your career by taking time for a residency, you will have to find one that meets your needs. You may realize quickly that your time is still not your own. You are earning more money, but you have bigger bills. If you have student loans, they have to be repaid. You may also have bought a house or car.

This is the time you need your colleagues the most. Schedule time to attend local and national professional association meetings. Get involved with a group of other new practitioners. Establish goals for your personal and professional life, and begin to take steps toward accomplishing them. This is the time in your life that you have been thinking about all through school. Now that it is here you need to take control.

Establishing Goals

It has been said that life is what happens to you when you're making other plans. For some people, life is what happens *because they aren't* making other plans. Establishing goals help you to achieve the kind of life you want. The first step is to examine each area of your life. Use the worksheets on pages 59, 60, 62, and 63 to help you define your priorities in life. You may want to post this list in a prominent place so that you can refer to it at least once a month. This will help you keep track of your goals and aid you in ascertaining your progress in reaching them.

Project Management

Goal setting and project management are intricately connected. Once a goal has been set, a plan of action must be established to reach the goal. People often fail to achieve their goals, not because their goals can't be achieved, but because they try to complete them all at once. You didn't complete your pharmacy training in a day, a week, a month, a semester, or even a year. You completed your training one course at a time, one day at a time, one semester at a time. Many of our personal and professional goals need to be viewed in the same way. By breaking goals into small, manageable, immediately achievable tasks, even the biggest goals can be accomplished. Consider using the worksheets on Reverse Stage Goal Setting[tm] (pages 63 and 64) to help you structure the accomplishment of your individual goals and to manage any project.

Staying Connected

Throughout this publication, we have stressed the importance of staying connected to and being actively involved in professional associations. At the beginning of your career, you need these connections more than ever.

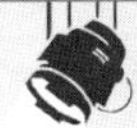

Long-Term Care

Dianne E. Tobias, Pharm.D.

President, Tobias Consulting Services

Dr. Dianne Tobias has owned and operated an independent consulting service specializing in geriatrics, quality improvement, data management, and educational programming since 1997. She has chosen to focus on long-term-care consulting but is also involved in a multi-consultant contract to provide interdisciplinary training at a Veterans Affair campus to various health care practitioners, including pharmacists. She has been the recipient of grants to study medication use in long-term care, assisted living, and dementia care settings in the United States and Canada. Consulting projects include developing and implementing a continuous quality improvement program, training, and strategic planning for a small chain of nursing and assisted living facilities, as well as home health and pharmacy clients. A long-term project has been to integrate therapeutic and adverse effect drug information to the *Resident Assessment Instrument*, a Health Care Financing Administration geriatric assessment tool used in all nursing facilities.

Dr. Tobias received her Pharm.D. degree from the University of California—San Francisco in 1971. At the beginning of her career, Dr. Tobias was an assistant professor of clinical pharmacy at the State University of New York School of Pharmacy and at the University of Maryland School of Pharmacy and a preceptor and assistant clinical professor of pharmacy at the University of California, Irvine. With other clinical and education faculty at the University of Maryland, Dr. Tobias developed patient simulation examinations for both B.S. and Pharm.D. students. This work led to jointly winning the Lyman Award from the American Association of Colleges of Pharmacy. Dr. Tobias became a consultant pharmacist in long-term-care settings in 1979. Dr. Tobias states, "Being a clinician in long-term care forced me to become more interdisciplinary and more global." She stresses the importance of communication and negotiation skills when discussing medication priorities with nonpharmacists.

Dr. Tobias joined a long-term-care company, and during her tenure of seventeen years, she served as a consultant, consultant director, quality assurance director of multiple disciplines, and quality improvement director of an entire nursing home chain. During this time, Dr. Tobias was appointed to the Joint Commission on Accreditation of Healthcare Organization's Long-term Care Professional and Technical Advisory Committee as a representa-

continued next page

Dianne E. Tobias, Pharm.D. *(continued)*

tive of ASCP. She was the first pharmacist representative to be appointed to this group and eventually became chair of the committee. Dr. Tobias states, "This experience showed me how global we need to be to optimally serve as patient advocates."

Dr. Tobias has been involved with professional associations throughout her career. Association involvement has meant a great deal to her both professionally and personally. She has been able to continue teaching by presenting at conferences and by publishing her work. Dr. Tobias has been a member of ASHP since graduation from pharmacy school and has been extensively involved with ASCP, just completing a term as its president. Dr. Tobias recommends new practitioners continue to hone their clinical skills, while developing skills in patient advocacy, communication, negotiating, and critical thinking. Dr. Tobias quotes, "Involvement breeds commitment. [My] work and involvement in associations have benefited me greatly by providing me with innumerable rewards and growth opportunities."

Professional associations help you learn about new techniques, legislation that impacts your work, continuing education that advances your knowledge, and contacts that will help you get your next job. Staying involved with associations gives you a voice and some influence in the growth and direction of the pharmacy profession.

Additionally, you need to stay connected on your job. Make allies at all levels. Never allow yourself to become isolated. Once you are out of the loop, you stop receiving the kind of inside information on which an organization runs. Gossip and office politics are things to avoid; but knowing the departmental budget, who has the ear of the director, and which projects are high profile will help you better manage your career.

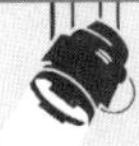

Long-Term Care

Jan Allen, R.Ph., FASCP

Vice President, National Accounts, GeriMed

Jan Allen is the Vice President of National Accounts for GeriMed, a long-term care group purchasing organization. She develops special programs for providers of long-term-care pharmacies. She works to increase and retain GeriMed's market share. She also provides educational opportunities and coordinates the efforts of the GeriMed Clinical Advisory Board. In addition to her position at GeriMed, Ms. Allen also has a private consulting business. She consults with nursing homes and presents educational training programs to pharmacists, nurses, long-term-care interdisciplinary staff, and others in the pharmaceutical industry. Although this type of work requires a great deal of travel, Ms. Allen is often able to work out of her home office.

Ms. Allen has worked in long-term care for over twenty years, beginning as a pharmacy student. When she made the decision to practice, her initial goal was a retail setting. It was only by chance that she was exposed to the long-term care arena, and she has loved the opportunities this has offered. After obtaining her degree from the Samford University McWhorter School of Pharmacy, Ms. Allen worked in a hospital setting and also gained some retail experience. Additionally, Ms. Allen has received leadership and other training in various programs, including a course in the Executive Program of Kellogg Graduate School of Management at Northwestern University.

Ms. Allen is a member of ASHP and has had extensive involvement with pharmacy organizations over the course of her career. She has held many offices—including president—with the American Society of Consultant Pharmacists (ASCP) and the Alabama Pharmacy Association. She is a member of the American Pharmaceutical Association, serving as an officer in the association's Academy of Pharmacy Practice and Management. She is also a member of the American Medical Directors Association. Additionally, Ms. Allen has held advisory board positions with the Alabama Medicaid Drug Utilization Review, Samford University McWhorter School of Pharmacy, Eli Lilly, Pfizer U.S. Pharmaceuticals Group, SmithKline Beecham, Rhône Poulenc Rorer, Parke-Davis, *Pharmacy Times* magazine, Novartis, Bayer, Roxanne, Glaxo Wellcome, and Forest.

Ms. Allen feels that being involved in varied organizations has been essential in establishing a unique practice. Her involvement in ASCP has been beneficial and a major contributor in the development of her practice. Being

continued next page

Jan Allen, R.Ph., FASCP *(continued)*

active in leadership enhanced her ability to take an active role in the long-term-care arena. In addition to her extensive activity with ASCP, she has also remained active in ASHP, APhA, AMDA, and APA. She has found ASHP meetings and exhibits to bring another viewpoint to her practice.

She also feels that it is very important to explore different avenues in the field of pharmacy. Ms. Allen states, "We have a great opportunity as well as an obligation to support our profession. We must remain active in our associations. This [includes] staying involved in the political process.... We must either make the rules or live with them. It is our choice, but more important, [it is] our obligation to protect and enhance our profession."

Components of a Complete Life

Listed below you will find eight major components of life that impact most of us. Many people don't often take the time to think about what they want to accomplish in their life or what will bring them satisfaction. Imagine that this is New Year's Eve 5, 10, and 20 years from now. You are reflecting on what you have accomplished in your life in the past. Write down what you see in each of these major areas.

Personal (e.g., time alone, playing, relaxation, personal development)

In 5 Years	In 10 Years	In 20 Years

Family (e.g., spouse/partner, children, others, home)

In 5 Years	In 10 Years	In 20 Years

Social (e.g., friends, group activities)

In 5 Years	In 10 Years	In 20 Years

Spiritual (e.g., religion, values, aesthetics, purpose, higher power)

In 5 Years	In 10 Years	In 20 Years

Financial (e.g., monetary goals, retirement planning, savings, big purchases)

In 5 Years	In 10 Years	In 20 Years

Intellectual (e.g., life time learning, certifications, advanced training)

In 5 Years	In 10 Years	In 20 Years

Professional (e.g., professional development, career goals, advancement)

In 5 Years	In 10 Years	In 20 Years

Societal (e.g., community involvement, charitable giving—time and money)

In 5 Years	In 10 Years	In 20 Years

Reverse-Stage Goal Setting™

"Where there is no vision the people perish."

1) Write your long-term goal below. This goal may be for the next year, next five years, or longer.

____

____

____

____

2) What must be accomplished immediately before completing the goal listed above:

____

____

3) What must be accomplished immediately before completing the goal listed in #2 above:

____

____

4) What must be accomplished immediately before completing the goal listed in #3 above:

____

____

5) What must be accomplished immediately before completing the goal listed in #4 above:

____

____

6) Continue to repeat this process until you can state a goal that can be reasonably started this month:

____

____

7) Now review the goal for this month and state the most important element of this goal that you can reasonably begin this week:

____

____

8) Now review the goal for this week and state the most important element of this goal that you can reasonably begin tomorrow:

____

____

9) Finally, review the goal for tomorrow and state the most important element of this goal that you can reasonably begin today:

____

____

10) Begin to accomplish the goal that you have set for today!!! Write your goals out; recite them; and review them daily.

"Setting goals tends to lead to success in reaching them."

Chapter 4

Personal Life Insight

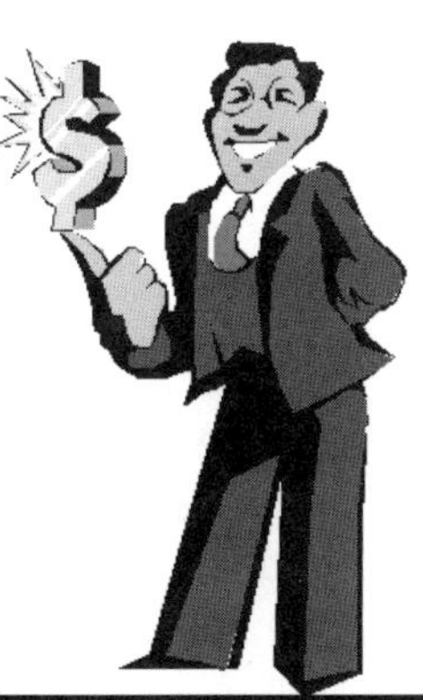

Note: The information provided in this section covers general financial planning, tax preparation, investing, and other particulars. ASHP makes no express or implied guarantees as to the accuracy or reliability of the information provided in this section. Each person's situation is different and financial, tax, and related information changes frequently. Not all of the options discussed in this chapter may be available to you or right for your needs. You should always consult an accountant, certified financial planner, investment broker, or other qualified professional to help you decide what is right for you.

Financial Planning

The following are a few common financial-related myths:

> *Myth #1: I need to repay my student loans before I save any other money.*

This really depends on several factors such as the amount you owe and the interest rate on it. A $10,000 loan at 5% annual interest costs less than a $7,000 loan at 9% annual interest. Furthermore, you will usually have a substantial amount of time (often 10 years) after graduation to pay back your loans. In the meantime, you should begin to set aside money for immediate needs and emergencies.

Myth #2: My employer has a retirement plan, so I don't need to invest any other money.

Your need to invest money is determined by such factors as the type of retirement plan, whether your employer contributes to the plan, and whether you are able to add to it. Consider how the employer plan is invested and how it has performed over the past 5, 10, and 20 years. Also, a retirement plan by definition is meant to set aside money for your retirement. You will need to save and invest money in plans you can access before you retire.

Myth #3: My retirement is at least 40 years from now. I can wait to begin investing.

Make no mistake about this: you need to begin investing as soon as you can. A 10% increase on a small investment each year for 40 years would grow exponentially, compared with a larger investment over 20, 25, or 30 years. Time matters in investing. The longer you give your money to grow, the more money you will get in return.

> Congress shall have the power to lay and collect taxes on income, from whatever source derived . . .
>
> —16th Amendment to the U.S. Constitution, ratified on February 25, 1913

Taxes

We all know Benjamin Franklin's famous statement that nothing is certain but death and taxes. Although the need to pay taxes is a certainty, we do have options in filing, paying, deferring, and (in some cases) legally avoiding taxes. Your individual tax liability is affected by your employment status (not whether you are employed, but rather who employs you). Are you self-employed? If so, are you a sole proprietor, an independent contractor, a partner, or self-employed in some other capacity? If you are an employee, you need to consider your withholding exemptions and whether you will be working part-time elsewhere. The tax withheld from your paycheck determines whether you will owe money or get a refund each year.

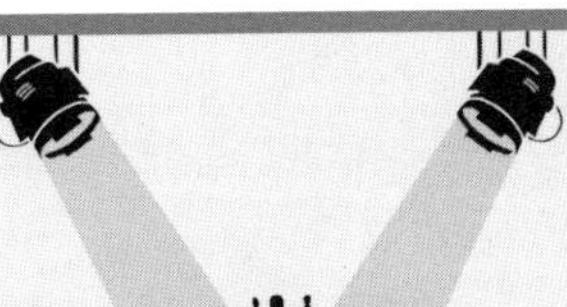

Practitioner Spotlight

Managed Care

Kent M. Nelson, Pharm.D., BCPS

Clinical Pharmacy Services Administrator, Kaiser Permanente Colorado Region
Assistant Professor (Adjoint)—University of Colorado School of Pharmacy

Dr. Kent Nelson has been the Clinical Pharmacy Services Administrator at Kaiser Permanente Colorado Region for three years. He supervises clinical pharmacy staff, is involved with staff recruiting, interacts with physician managers, identifies opportunities to improve patient outcomes through disease state management, and oversees the formulary. His other duties include budget preparation, quality assurance, strategizing future clinical pharmacy opportunities, and justifying additional clinical pharmacy positions.

Dr. Nelson received his Pharm.D. at the University of Texas. While completing the coursework for his Pharm.D., he spent three years working in hospital pharmacies. He completed an internal medicine residency at University Hospital in San Antonio, Texas. Dr. Nelson worked for four years as a clinical pharmacy specialist in internal medicine at a Kaiser Permanente medical office. He feels this experience helped him appreciate the challenges facing primary care physicians and sharpened his patient care and communication skills. He also worked some evenings in the outpatient pharmacy and believes this has helped him understand the challenges facing pharmacists in the Kaiser Permanente outpatient pharmacies.

Dr. Nelson has been involved with ASHP in a variety of ways. He has served on the Commission on Therapeutics since 1998 and has facilitated a focus group on telepharmacy. He has spoken at national and state meetings and believes this networking provides him with innovative ideas for new clinical pharmacy services.

Dr. Nelson explains that new practitioners need to understand the current marketplace. He looks for practitioners with flexibility and excellent communication skills. He asks, "Can you market your drug therapy expertise to physicians, nurses, and patients?" New practitioners must be able to work collaboratively in interdisciplinary teams. He questions, "Do you understand the goals of your patients and the organization?" He expresses that an individual's interpersonal skills will provide the opportunities to use clinical skills. In order to be successful, Dr. Nelson believes that new practitioners must be willing to practice in environments that may differ from that of their academic training.

continued next page

Kent M. Nelson, Pharm.D., BCPS *(continued)*

Dr. Nelson concludes, "With the national pharmacist shortage, some new practitioners are tempted by rising salaries to complete their training quickly. Although on-the-job training is useful, do not underestimate the value of residency and fellowship training. Although your future salary levels may not exceed that of your colleagues, the skills that you can develop will allow you to effectively compete for the position you desire."

> There is only one thing worse than the flu season: the tax season. You can recover from the flu.
>
> —Unknown

People have different philosophies about what constitutes success in filing their taxes. Some are happy if they get a large refund; others prefer to owe money (on the belief that they have gotten to use the money during the year). Relying on a refund check may not be a good idea because it keeps you from being in charge of your income and taxes. Owing a significant amount when you file is also not a good idea, for the same reason. The best situation would be to work with an accountant to plan ahead so that you are paying out (either in withholding or estimated quarterly payments to the federal, state, and local governments) only what you owe. Getting a small refund or owing a small amount each year keeps you in control and allows you to plan better your spending and saving.

> I am proud to be paying taxes in the United States. The only thing is—I could be just as proud for half the money.
>
> —Arthur Godfrey

Retirement Planning and Investing

Investing and retirement planning are personal choices that should be made on the basis of your income and expenses now and your expectations for the future. Some financial planners may tell you that you should save a percentage of every paycheck and consistently pay yourself (via your savings or investments) first and then pay your bills. Or you may choose to

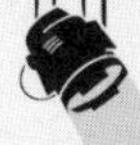
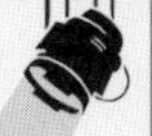

Managed Care

Darlene M. Mednick, M.B.A., R.Ph., PAHN, NPDP

Vice President, Pharmacy Relations, Merck-Medco Managed Care

Darlene Mednick has worked in managed care pharmacy for fifteen years. At present, she cultivates relationships with both colleges of pharmacy and professional pharmacy organizations and provides strategic leadership for pharmacist recruitment. She facilitates training and education to increase awareness and understanding of Merck-Medco and the opportunities that exist for pharmacists within managed care or pharmacy benefit management companies.

Ms. Mednick has experienced a variety of practice settings. She worked in community pharmacy practice for eight years and in nursing home consulting for more than a year. Her managed care practice experience is vast, including six years with a group-model health maintenance organization, more than four years at a national independent practice association insurer, and more than four years as a pharmacy benefit manager.

Ms. Mednick has been an active participant in ASHP activities by contributing to membership publications, educational materials, and ASHP meetings and programming. She has been a speaker during ASHP meetings, represented residency programs in the ASHP Residency Showcase, and cultivated staff relationships, which have resulted in ASHP program involvement.

Ms. Mednick offers the following advice to new practitioners, "Explore exciting career opportunities in managed care—it's not a nontraditional or alternative practice setting any more!" She encourages new practitioners to commit to lifelong learning and be open to continual learning and growth. She stresses the importance of acquiring important life skills including project management and communications skills, such as writing, verbal presentation, and listening. She also mentions the importance of the following skills for a new practitioner: relationship building, teamwork and collaboration, negotiation, conflict management, and meeting facilitation including group decision-making models.

Ms. Mednick encourages new practitioners to be realistic in the level of their first job after school. Although the Pharm.D. degree is important, she believes it does not replace the time and skills required to develop appropriate management skills. She encourages new practitioners to find ways to develop management and leadership skills. Get involved in professional pharmacy associations and actively contribute, she advises.

save a fixed amount or fund your retirement account once a year. Whatever method you choose, saving is important to your financial health and future.

A myriad of plans exist, ranging from savings accounts to personal investment to individual tax-deferred accounts to employer-sponsored retirement plans. A very brief overview of some options is presented below.

401(k) Plans. With 401(k) plans, employees may invest a portion of their salary in a tax-sheltered savings account set up by their employer. There is a limit on how much can be invested in a 401(k) each year, but it is often above the $2000 individual retirement account (IRA) cap. Many companies offering 401(k) plans match part of the employee's contribution. Matching contributions do not count toward the annual cap, but if you quit your job after just a few years (as designated by employers), you may forfeit all or part of the matching deposits.

Company Pension and Profit-Sharing Plans. If you work for a company that offers a pension or profit-sharing program, you should review the plan's information with your accountant, tax advisor, or financial planner. Many companies offer generous plans; however, you need to understand all of the terms and rules involved. For instance, penalties often apply if you take money out of a company plan early. Since the money in a retirement plan is meant to be used after a person retires, such a penalty is designed to encourage you to roll over early payouts into an IRA.

IRAs. You can contribute up to $2000 per year to an IRA if the earned income is at least equal to the amount contributed. All, some, or none of that $2000 may be tax deductible depending on your income and tax filing status. However, a deductible IRA cannot be established by individuals who participate in various other retirement plans. Contributions to an IRA can be made for any year in which you have earned income until you reach the age of 70½. Also, if you are income eligible, IRAs can be partially or fully converted to Roth IRAs (see below). IRAs can be funded with stocks, bonds, bank certificates of deposits (CDs), various mutual funds, and annuities. Dividends, interest, and capital gain growth within traditional IRAs are generally not taxable until money is withdrawn. Withdrawals before age 59½ may be subject to taxes and an IRS penalty.

Roth IRAs. Like with traditional IRAs, an individual may contribute up to $2000 a year to the Roth IRA, but this money is not tax deductible. Asset growth, dividends, and interest are not taxed in the Roth IRA, and money withdrawn from the plan is tax free under certain conditions. Most individuals can establish a Roth IRA if their income is below a certain threshold, and can still participate even if enrolled in various other retirement plans.

SEP-IRAs. Any business can establish a SEP-IRA for their employees.

Practice Management

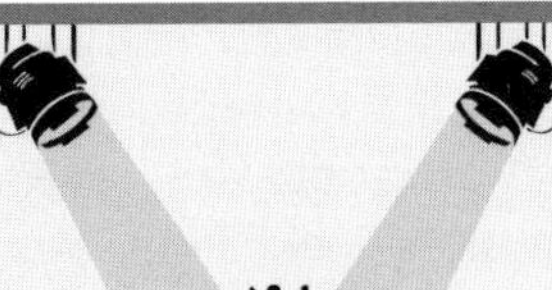

Jane S. Henry, M.B.A., R.Ph., FASHP

Director of Pharmacy, St. Francis Hospital and Medical Center

Jane Henry has worked in pharmacy practice management for twenty years. Her duties include hiring and firing, budget preparation and adherence, working with other departments outside of the pharmacy to facilitate changes, performance improvement reporting for the pharmacy, and planning for the future direction of the department. Her staff includes an inpatient pharmacy supervisor and a medical building retail pharmacy supervisor.

Ms. Henry has been a very active member of ASHP. She has attended nearly every ASHP Midyear Clinical Meeting since 1979 and most ASHP Annual Meetings since the early 1980's. She has served in the ASHP House of Delegates as a member and chair of the Committee on Nominations for three years, as a member of the Council on Administrative Affairs, and a member of the Board of Directors from 1995 to 1998. She is currently involved with the ASHP Practice Change Model.

Ms. Henry states, "How could I have accomplished anything in my practice without my ASHP involvement? [ASHP] has afforded me the opportunity to meet and get to know many of the profession's leaders with whom I have been in contact at various times for information or advice."

When hiring, Ms. Henry looks for three things that differentiate successful candidates from others: a positive attitude, a patient focus, and membership in professional organizations. She encourages new practitioners, "You get out of pharmacy what you put into it! If you are sincere and committed to making the lives of your patients better, it will shine through. While every day offers its challenges, maintaining a positive focus and being open to new ideas is essential if we hope to have the profession progress and be able to use our skills and knowledge to improve the lives of our patients."

An employer can restrict participation in the SEP-IRA on the basis of certain criteria. However, once an employee is deemed eligible, contributions to each individual's retirement account must be allocated in a non-discriminatory manner. Contributions to an SEP-IRA come directly from the employer, can vary from year to year, and can be discontinued at any time and for any reason—but they must be discontinued for all employees. Self-employed individuals can contribute a maximum of 13.04% of their net self-employment income to the plan.

Stocks and Mutual Funds. Stocks are investments in a company. Shares of stock represent your percent ownership of that company based on the total amount of shares offered by the company. If a company has 1000 shares of stock and you own 100 shares, then you own 10% of the company. Most companies have from hundreds of thousands to millions of shares of stock. Investing in the stock market is a very serious business, and it is usually best to work with a professional in picking stocks and investing your money. Over a substantial period of time (5, 10, 20 years), values of shares in major companies have seen a 10–20% growth. As a result, for the average person investing in the stock market should be seen as a long-term strategy for increasing wealth.

Since owning a few shares in a few companies requires much longer to achieve any substantial growth, investment firms have established mutual funds. Money from many investors is pooled in order to own larger blocks of stock in many companies. This helps the fund weather the daily ups and downs in prices of individual companies. Many financial planners recommend that investors new to the stock market consider a mutual fund as a first step. There are many different funds to suit a variety of investors. Funds may focus on growth, stability, technology, health care, small companies, large companies, etc. Some funds charge fees to invest; others allow you to invest even as little as $50 a month without a fee.

Short-Term vs. Long-Term Investments. Once you invest in a qualified retirement plan, your money will grow tax free until you withdraw it. Because you would have to pay taxes and a large penalty if you withdraw before a defined age (usually 59½), retirement savings are a long-term investment. This means that you need to anticipate each year how much you can afford to save, because you will lose a lot more if you withdraw it early.

Short-term investing is encouraged for special projects and quick returns on investments. For instance, if you have $500 that you won't need immediately but expect to need within a few months, you might consider a CD. Or you could purchase stock in a stable company that pays a dividend (i.e., 10%) each year. The stock may not go up much in value while you own it, but the dividend pays a higher interest rate than it will in a bank account that pays only 2 or 3% interest.

Student Loans

Repayment Options. There are several typical student loan repayment options. The standard repayment option requires that you make combined principal and interest payments each month throughout the loan repay-

Practice Management

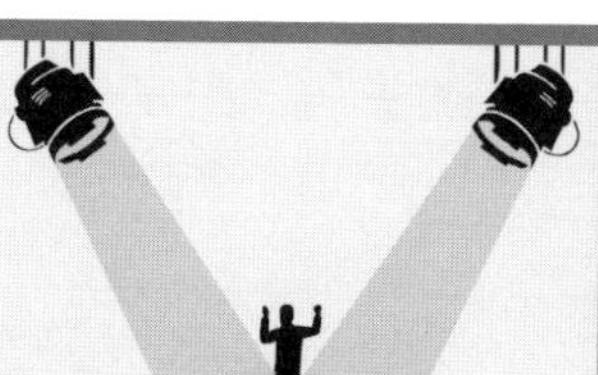

Joseph T. Botticelli, M.S., R.Ph.

Director of Pharmacy and Rehabilitation Services, St. Joseph Medical Center

Joseph Botticelli has been the Director of Pharmacy at St. Joseph Medical Center since 1996 and in the expanded role with Rehabilitation Services since 1997. In Rehabilitation Services, he develops new programs, reviews the overall performance of the department, and works on budget development. In the pharmacy, Mr. Botticelli evaluates current and proposed services, supports the orientation and training of staff, and establishes performance improvement mechanisms. With both departments, he represents the staff at administrative and clinical meetings, such as the Pharmacy and Therapeutics Committee, Performance Improvement, and Joint Commission Preparedness.

Mr. Botticelli states, "I have been blessed with quite a number and variety of pharmacy mentors. They all contributed to my development as a pharmacy leader." His first significant pharmacy experience was as a technician at the University of Wisconsin Hospital and Clinics. He learned about residency programs and the value these programs bring to career development. After a yearlong internship and a two-year residency program, he worked at Rush–Presbyterian St. Luke's Medical Center in Chicago, Illinois. He served as Coordinator of Drug Systems in addition to some of the centralized services and later managed some of the inpatient pharmacy satellites. Later, he took the position of Assistant Director of Pharmacy at the Medical University of South Carolina and served as a faculty member in the College of Pharmacy before taking on his current roles.

Mr. Botticelli has served in many capacities for ASHP and its state affiliates. He has participated in the Information Network for Students program for ASHP and served on the Council on Administrative Affairs (1998–2000). He feels these opportunities have afforded him the chance to think about pharmacy at a very high policy level rather than a local or state level.

Mr. Botticelli feels we are in an unprecedented, opportunity-filled time in the pharmacy profession's history. New and more-seasoned practitioners must take advantage of these opportunities and expand the role of pharmacy throughout the continuum of each patient's health care. He states, "Keep learning through residency, certification, and other training programs as well as ongoing continuing education. New practitioners cannot limit their edu-

continued next page

Joseph T. Botticelli, M.S., R.Ph. *(continued)*

cation to their schools and colleges of pharmacy. Stay involved!" Mr. Botticelli concludes, "The role of a pharmacist in any practice setting is what you make of it. It is very easy to slide into the comfort zone and merely respond to physician orders. You turn into a robot, devoid of all thinking. It is much harder to keep those ideals that are learned in pharmacy school. Never give up! It is those that work hard for the patient that succeed."

ment term. Graduated repayment plans allow for smaller initial monthly payments and increase at set periods during the term of the loan. As the name implies, income-based repayment schedules are monthly payments based on a percentage of the borrower's monthly gross income. Some borrowers may qualify for extended repayment that provides a lengthened repayment term of up to 25 years. Loan deferment options vary, depending on the kind of loans you have. A deferment is a temporary suspension of loan payments for specific situations, such as attending school at least half-time, being unemployed (time limited), studying in an approved graduate fellowship or rehabilitation program for the disabled, or experiencing economic hardship (time limited). If you have any trouble paying your education loans, contact your loan servicer immediately. Being proactive and honest about your situation will help you get the assistance you need. To determine if you qualify for any change in a repayment schedule or deferment, contact you loan counselor or financial advisor.

Loan Consolidation and Serialization. Loan consolidation allows the borrower to refinance multiple loans. In this scenario, the original loans are paid off and a new loan for the total combined balance of the previous loans is created. Typically the new loan will have a new term, a new repayment schedule, and many times, a new (sometimes lower) interest rate. Loan serialization is similar to consolidation. Your loans are purchased from other institutions and then serviced by the new buyer in one account. You would make one monthly payment, but keep the original terms and interest rates of the individual loans.

To see what your monthly payments might be, take advantage of Sallie Mae's repayment calculator (http://www.salliemae.com/calculators/repayment.html).

Home—Renting vs. Buying

Many of you have spent much, if not all, of your post high school education living in a dormitory or apartment. Now that you are out of school, working, and earning more money than you likely have ever earned, you are considering whether you should continue renting or should buy a home. There are differing opinions about whether it is financially better to rent or buy. Some of the issues to consider include your current financial situation (i.e., how much debt you have, how much money you have saved, your monthly expenses), your living and working situations (i.e., whether you plan to live or work in a particular location more than three years), your short- and long-term goals, and your investment and retirement strategies.

Live the Dream—Buy Your Home. When considering what to do, many ask themselves "Can I afford to buy?" A better question to ask may be "Can I afford to continue renting?" When you write a check each month for your apartment, that money is *gone*. You build up no equity and when you leave, all you get back (maybe) is the security deposit. When you buy a house, however, each month's mortgage check gets you closer to ownership. If you move, you will get not only the equity you built up but, in many cases, an increase in the value of the home itself. It usually requires several years to see an appreciation of the investment, however. Also, once you lock in the interest rate and payment schedule, your payments stay the same. Your salary, however, is likely to increase over time. The result is that your mortgage payment becomes a smaller and smaller percentage of your overall income. Rent payments, on the other hand, tend to increase with inflation and may keep pace with increases in your paycheck.

There are other advantages to being a homeowner; for example, property taxes and interest payments on a mortgage for an owner-occupied home are currently tax-deductible. In the early years of a typical mortgage, all but a small percentage of each monthly payment goes toward paying the interest on the loan. Deducting the payments you make on property taxes and mortgage payments will reduce your annual taxable income. Later, as you increase the equity in your home, you may choose to take out a home equity loan. Currently, the interest on up to $100,000 of home equity indebtedness is tax deductible.

Another tax advantage relates to appreciation in the value of your home. When you sell your home for more than you originally paid, the gain in home value is not taxable if you purchase another home for a price equal to or greater than the sale price of the home you sold. Once you're past age 55 when you sell your home, even if you do not purchase another home of equal or greater value, you can currently recognize a tax-free gain of up to $120,000.

Be Flexible—Rent Your Home. People choose to rent for various personal reasons such as limited cash, uncertainty about location and availability of work or living arrangements, a busy lifestyle, and a desire for flexibility. Depending on your lifestyle, age, and financial situation, some advisors may encourage renting rather than buying. When choosing a home or apartment to rent, you should consider the initial expense of moving in (security deposit, first and last month's rent, rental insurance), the level of privacy and noise, safety of the location, and the ease with which you can terminate your lease.

Buying a home means a higher level of financial and personal commitment needed for upkeep and repairs, such as painting, lawn maintenance, and cleaning rain gutters. Also, the cost of buying includes more than the monthly mortgage. The typical costs of buying consist of a minimum down payment of 5% of the total purchase price; legal fees; transfer tax; home inspection and appraisal; home and mortgage insurance; various application fees, property taxes; water, sewer, and utility adjustments; hook-up fees for cable, telephone, and power; and other moving and miscellaneous expenses. All of these costs add up and can mean paying $10,000–$15,000 before you can move in. In addition to these up-front costs, a mortgage is usually higher than monthly rent. If you saved and invested, for example, $500 a month and earned 8% interest over a period of 20 years, you would have a savings of over $250,000. Although real estate has traditionally increased in value, it hasn't reached these levels for the average homeowner.

Your Car—Buying vs. Leasing

It wouldn't be surprising if you have never bought a new car. While in school, many students need help just to pay for school and living expenses. Once new graduates find a job, however, the temptation may be to go out and make their first big purchase—a new car. This may seem like an exciting opportunity, but it might not be the best decision. There are actually two issues that need to be addressed. The first is buying a new versus a used car. The second is whether you should buy a car or lease it.

New Car or Used. Most of us like the idea of owning new things. We rarely buy used clothes, and leftover tuna casserole has become a national joke. So it isn't any wonder that owning a new car is seen as desirable. If you plan to use a car at least five years and drive it more than 15,000 miles a year, then a new car might be a good idea. Be sure to check the model's safety, service, and performance record, and consider buying an extended warranty. If you are spending $20,000 or more for a new car, you want to be certain that maintenance and other costs are kept to a minimum. Also, comparison shop for the best deals on the make and model you want and the best interest rate for financing (the Internet can be of great help here). Depending on the car and the dealership and your credit record, you may be able to finance a new car for less than 2%. In addition, the best times to buy a new car are during the middle of the week, at the end of the month, and after the next year's models have been introduced. Most people buy new cars on the weekend (when they have time to go). At the end of the month sales people and dealerships are eager to increase their sales figures and are more willing to make deals. When the next year's models are introduced, there is a big push to clear last year's inventory. Finally, *never* buy on impulse or at the first dealership you visit. Shop around, and let the dealer know that you are looking for the best deal. You may go back to the first dealership, but you need to be an educated buyer. Don't be afraid to *think* about a deal. There is nothing worse than realizing too late that you could have bought more car for less money.

But before you buy a new car, consider this: many financial advisors say that buying a new car is the worst investment you can make. The reason is that depreciation and interest often account for more than half the cost of owning and operating a car. Within three years, most new cars will be worth less than half of what they cost new. However, not all cars age equally; some cars lose value faster than others. After all, depreciation is a function of supply and demand, and this can create bargains for used-car buyers. Even a year-old car will be worth less then, and, by shopping around, you might find the best deal.

Owning a new car is attractive, and there will likely come a time in your life when it is a better decision. However, if you drive less than 15,000 miles a year, buying a used car is a better choice now. You may find that saving your money, paying off student loans, or investing helps you more at this time in your life.

Buying vs. Leasing. Whether you are considering a new or used car, you may have the option of leasing. About one-third of all new car drivers are leasing their vehicles. Leasing typically means lower up-front and monthly costs, which often means that you can get a more expensive car than if you purchased it outright. If you choose to lease, you will likely get a new (or newer) car every two or three years. You don't have to worry about trade-in value, and depending on the package you get, you might not have to be bothered with maintenance. If you drive fewer than 12,000 miles a year, leasing *might* be a good option.

However, there are other financial factors to consider: first there are often additional fees to contend with, including capitalized cost reduction (a down payment); security deposits, set-up fee, and service contracts; finance charges, rent charge, or interest rate; excess mileage (anything over a minimum yearly mileage beginning as low as 12,000 miles) and wear fees; monthly sales or use taxes; gap insurance (insurance that pays the difference between what you owe and what your insurance covers when your vehicle is damaged beyond repair); disposition fee (a fee at the end of some lease agreements if you decide to return the car rather than buy it); and early cancellation fees. These can all add up and need to be reviewed carefully. However, fees are usually negotiable, so don't sign without pushing for a better deal. Finally, carefully consider how long the lease term is in months and what the *actual* monthly payments will be. If you plan to lease more than 30 months, you might be able to buy a car for not much more than what you will pay to lease one.

Remember, if there is a deal in owning a car, it occurs when the car's usefulness is longer than the payments you make. If you keep a car for ten years, at least five should be payment-free. When you lease, you never drive for free. If you drive a lot, aren't particular about what you drive, or plan to pass your car on to your child, leasing isn't your best option. Before agreeing to any lease, read the contract at home with a friend or relative and calculate the total cost.

Job Benefit Evaluation

When considering a job offer, people typically focus on such factors as salary, location, and prestige. These are certainly important, but there are other things that you have already indicated are important to your job satisfaction. Go back to chapter 1, and review your Work-Life Factors Summary on pages 23 and 24 to see how closely the job you are considering matches the factors you listed as important. Use this list each time you are interviewed.

In addition to salary, the benefits package (leave time, health insurance, professional development, etc.) is one of the areas people cite as important in choosing a job. And, when people complain about their job and when they look to change, their benefits package is often a huge reason for staying or moving on. Two areas of benefits new pharmacists should study in any job offer evaluation include health insurance and professional liability coverage.

Health Insurance. Health insurance coverage of some kind is generally included in almost all full-time employment settings. If the company or organization makes health coverage available, then it will likely be available to all employees who meet certain criteria. For instance, coverage may be limited to full-time employees, to employees who have been with the organization a certain period of time (usually 90 days), or to employees, but not independent contractors.

When evaluating health insurance plans, find out what the enrollment criteria are. Also, ask whether or not there are any limits to participating in the employer's health insurance plan. If there are multiple plans to choose from, you need to review them carefully and decide on the basis of your lifestyle, health conditions, and financial situation. You would choose the plan that best addresses your needs, such as selecting your own physician, or if you are planning on getting married or having a child. There are several types of health insurance plans available; however, not all types may be offered by each employer.

Traditional Indemnity Insurance. In this type of plan, you can receive services from any doctor or hospital of your choice. You will typically have to file claim forms to receive reimbursement for out-of-pocket expenses and you may not receive coverage for preventive care. In one type of indemnity insurance, costs are controlled by requiring prior approval for hospitalization and certain outpatient procedures; but you can still choose any doctor and have access to any hospital.

Health Maintenance Organizations (HMOs). Although there are different types of HMOs, they have similarities. Each person insured by an HMO chooses a primary care physician from a specific network of doctors. Every time the person goes to a doctor other than this physician, a referral must be granted from the primary care doctor in advance, even for covered treatment by a specialist who is part of the HMO. Generally, referrals are not needed in emergency situations. Typically HMOs have no deductibles to meet (although there may be upper limits on coverage), but there are copayments that must be made when seeking services. Preventive care is usually a standard part of the coverage, and there are usually no forms to fill out.

The first type of HMO is the group model. In this format, services are offered from contracted hospitals or salaried physicians at the HMO's own medical centers. Patients who use this type of HMO usually must use the HMO's medical center doctors and hospitals.

The second type of HMO is the independent practice association. This type of HMO is similar to the group model except that in this plan the HMO contracts with individual physicians who care for plan members in their private offices. These physicians are free to work with more than one plan and usually offer care on a fee-for-service basis as well.

The third type of HMO is the point-of-service plan. In this type of plan, services can be obtained from any doctor or hospital, but copayments are lower if network providers are used. Additional paperwork may be required to get approval for some services.

Preferred Provider Organizations (PPOs). PPOs combine elements of traditional indemnity insurance and HMOs. Like HMOs, PPOs have networks of physicians and hospitals that discount their rates for individuals participating in the plan. But, unlike HMOs, not all PPOs use or require a specific primary care physician to oversee a member's overall care. Members can see a specialist whenever they feel it is necessary. Members are strongly encouraged to see network physicians by being reimbursed less if they go outside the network for treatment. There may be additional paperwork to get approval for some services, and preventive care may not always be covered.

Deductibles are another feature common to many PPO plans. Before the member is eligible for the maximum reimbursement benefit, he or she must pay all of the costs up to the deductible amount. Additionally, many PPO plans include a coinsurance feature. For example, if the plan has a $5,000 coinsurance component, once the deductible is met, the member will receive a 100% reimbursement after the member reaches $5,000 in medical bills.

Once you know the type of plans offered by the company and their eligibility requirements, you must choose what best meets your needs. First, even if you are not eligible to participate in the company's plan because you are an independent contractor you may negotiate with the organization to be included at your own expense. Buying into a group plan may be cheaper than finding coverage on your own. If you aren't eligible and can't buy into the health insurance plan, then you might negotiate for the cash equivalent of the insurance premium so that you can buy your own coverage. In fact, even if you are eligible to participate in an existing plan, you may request cash toward an insurance plan of your own choosing. If none of the plans offered by the company meets your needs, you may negotiate with the employer to give the cash they would be spending on your coverage either to you or to a plan of your choosing and you would pay the difference.

Liability Coverage. As a pharmacist, you will need professional liability insurance so that you are covered in the event a patient sues you. Whether you are an employee or an independent contractor, you should ask your employer the extent to which you are *personally* covered in the event of a lawsuit. In many cases, a lawsuit will name not only the organization but also any practitioner involved in the situation. The organization will almost certainly have liability insurance covering the business, but that coverage may or may not extend to individual employees and contractors.

If your employer tells you that you are covered, you should request documentation. Consider having an attorney review this to determine if you need additional protection. If you are advised to obtain private liability coverage, shop around. Start your research with your professional association. Associations have often negotiated excellent group rates, and you can usually get first-rate coverage at the lowest possible price. When applying, discuss with the insurance company representatives why you are seeking coverage, and ask them to recommend the right policy. You may be able to buy insurance that covers any gap between what the employer's policy covers and what you need. Another option is to find out who provides the coverage for your company and to discuss with them a policy that would cover your work with that organization. Also speak with other pharmacists as they may have insights about the type and limits of coverage that might be best for you.

Salary and Benefits Negotiation

We reviewed health and liability insurance above, as they are key areas with which many new practitioners may be unfamiliar. But, when evaluating a job offer, it is important to remember that almost *everything* is negotiable: salary, benefits, start date, vacation time, etc. The following are a few guidelines to make your negotiation more successful:

Timing. There is an old saying, "The person who mentions money first, loses." When interviewing for a job, you should try to deflect questions about your salary and benefits expectations *until* the potential employer commits to you. Once you are offered the position, you have leverage. Until then, you are just another applicant. If possible, when you are asked about salary, ask the interviewers what amount has been budgeted for the position. Most of the time they won't tell you, but if they do, you have the upper hand. Usually, any figure they give you has some room to move up.

Understand the Offer. The next step in effective negotiation is to understand the offer. Are there any contingencies? When do you have to make a decision? Are you being offered a one-year contract or an open-ended one? What does the offer include (e.g., salary, leave time, health insurance, a signing bonus)? Once you know what is being offered and when you need to respond, you will be in a better position to evaluate the offer.

Know Your Market Value. As mentioned before, an article in USA *Today* reported that starting salaries for new pharmacy graduates ranged from $67,000 to $75,000. According to the article, some employers are offering signing bonuses and expensive cars. Through networking, informational interviewing, association salary surveys, online searches, and job offers, you will begin to discover what the market says your skills and knowledge are worth. This is vital. You must know what the typical salary, benefits, and other perks are so that when an offer is made you will know whether it is higher or lower than average or on target.

Know Your Bottom Line. Regardless of what is being offered or what the typical level of compensation is, you need to know what you will accept. People often say that money isn't everything, but when negotiating a salary, that is often all they think about. Sometimes an employer has no flexibility on salary and benefits. However, if pushed, the employer may be able to grant a flexible work schedule, more leave time, paid conference participation, or any number of non-monetary perks. Also, if you know that you must have a certain level of income to be able to pay your bills, then you can't accept an offer below that figure.

Know When to Walk Away. Without this ability, you cannot negotiate. If you can't turn down an offer for any reason, then you can't negotiate. If you have done your homework, know what you are worth, know what you want, and are offered a job that you want but at a level of compensation below what you expect, then you have two choices: accept or negotiate. If you attempt to negotiate, it is possible that the employer will say that there is no flexibility. It is also possible that the offer will be withdrawn (although the employer is more likely to say, "We will be in touch" and then not call you until someone else has accepted the offer).

If you see no flexibility in the employer's position, then you either have to accept their offer or walk away. If you walk away, the employer may call you back to negotiate or find someone else. Often the employer will look for someone else. If that were to occur, you must keep in mind that you would not have been satisfied if you had accepted an offer below what you know to be legitimate for someone in your field, living and working in your area, and with your level of skills and education.

Family

Work is an important part of life, but it isn't all there is to life. Regardless of gender and lifestyle, you have a need for personal time and for a life with your family—those who are closest and most important to you. There are some options that you may want to consider, especially if you decide to have children or if you care for aging parents or for a spouse who needs physical care because of an illness or other special need.

Job Sharing. You may consider working part-time with someone who shares your needs or desires for a limited work schedule. Job sharing is a special form of part-time work where two people of equivalent education and skill share the duties and responsibilities of one full-time job. The salary and benefits are often also split equally (although some employers may increase the percentage of health insurance benefits above 50%). In order for this plan to work effectively, you must have an employer who is open to the idea and find a job-share partner who has similar work habits and ethics. If your employer agrees, you may need to work more than 20 hours a week for both job-share partners to attend staff meetings or have overlap time.

Read an article at WomensWire.com (http://more.womenswire.com/myths/share.html) to gain more insight on job sharing. Although job sharing is not only for women, women tend to make up a greater percentage of those who participate. Another Web site that you might find helpful is http://www.mommd.com/jobshare/. This site is for physicians who are also mothers and, while not specifically geared to pharmacists, may provide insights on medical professionals who job share.

Job Flexibility. Related to job sharing is job flexibility. Instead of splitting time with other professionals, pharmacists with a flexible job schedule work 40 hours a week in any combination that fits their schedule and their employer's needs. For instance, they might work four 10-hour days and have one week day off, or nine 9-hour days (four 9-hour days in week one, with Friday off and five 9-hour days in week two). Or they may have the opportunity to work less than 40 hours in one week by giving notice to their employer or by having someone else fill in. In most cases this would mean getting paid less for the week or month in which they worked less than a full-time schedule.

The point is to be able to make the job work around your life and needs rather than the other way around. This plan usually requires an understanding and flexible employer and some level of respect within the organization so that an employer will trust that this flexibility will not be abused. If possible, job flexibility can make the difference between keeping a good job or having to take PRN shift work.

Family Friendly Employment. Even before the Family and Medical Leave Act became law in 1993, many people were talking about family friendly employment. In fact, different magazines (e.g., Working Woman, workingwoman.com) rate the most family friendly employers. Family friendly employment means different things to different people, but it typically implies that an employer understands the needs of employees to have work that supports their family life and may help with child and elder care. These employers may have onsite daycare; provide a stipend for day or elder care; provide paid maternity and paternity leave; have an employee who assists with child care, elder care, school choice, and other such issues; and have flexible work and leave schedules.

Stress Management

No matter what occurs in your work or personal life, you will experience stress. Most psychologists agree that there are two types of stress and that we need a balance of stress in our lives in order to succeed. Eustress is positive stress; it energizes, motivates, and excites us. Distress is negative stress; it overloads, provides pain, and wears down on us. If we have enough stress in our life, we are optimally productive. If we have too little or too much stress, we are either bored or overwhelmed. Coping with stress, stress management, means understanding and learning how to work with it.

First, you need to recognize your "stress triggers"—things that set you off and tend to lead to stress in your life. If you can avoid or minimize contact with these stress triggers, you will be better able to deal with the stress in your life.

Next, understand how long you have to deal with the stress. Knowing the duration of the stressful event or situation often helps people cope. Even if it will last a long time, understanding that it will end (and knowing approximately when) has enabled people to endure many difficult circumstances.

Also, it is important to have people who support and encourage you. Thinking about your strengths and support system is a good way to deal with the stress in your life. If you know that a stressful event or situation is coming and you know who is available to help you cope, you will typically manage your stress better.

Finally, learning and building on your unique coping strategies will help you manage stress rather than be controlled by it. Some hints for better stress management include making changes in small steps rather than all at once; having clear, concrete, and specific goals; rewarding yourself periodically so that you feel compensated; having who understands what you are going through and who will listen when you complain; and learning to affirm yourself daily—positive self-talk aimed at keeping your spirits up.

Chapter 5

Using ASHP as a Professional Development Resource

Education

ASHP has an excellent reputation for providing high quality, current pharmacist education. Educational programs at meetings, special conferences, online resources, and print publications bring ASHP members the most up-to-date information on therapeutic and administrative pharmacy practice topics.

ASHP Meetings. Members receive reduced registration rates when attending ASHP's national meetings, the Annual Meeting, and the Midyear Clinical Meeting. The opportunities for professional development at these meetings are numerous, including educational programs, contributed paper and poster sessions, workshops, and networking. Many members believe that networking with colleagues is the best part of belonging to ASHP. Through ASHP, its meetings, and fifty state affiliate societies, a pharmacist's opportunity to make professional contacts is unlimited.

ASHP Midyear Clinical Meeting. The Midyear Clinical Meeting takes place every December and is the largest meeting dedicated to improving patient care through drug therapy in the world. Over 20,000 attendees take part in more than seventy educational programs highlighting current therapeutic and administrative pharmacy practice trends. A variety of activities exist for practitioners, including more than 1,000 contributed papers and posters, specialist networking forums, pre-meeting workshops, student programming, an extensive exhibit hall displaying the latest technologies and products, the Residency Showcase, and the Personnel Placement Service.

The Residency Showcase is an excellent opportunity to learn about ASHP-accredited residency programs. Attendees have a chance to meet current residents and preceptors and gain information about their programs and institutions. The showcase primarily focuses on pharmacy practice residencies; however, programs that also offer specialty residencies might offer information on both types of residencies at the exhibit. The list of participating programs is published in the October 15 issue of the *AJHP*. It is also important to get a copy of each day's newspaper to look for any changes. If you plan to attend the Residency Showcase, consider signing up for the Residency Match during the fall to review some programs before attending the meeting. For those new practitioners interested in pursuing a specialty residency, the Personnel Placement Service is the most appropriate venue.

ASHP Annual Meeting. The ASHP Annual Meeting takes place every June and attracts more than 5,000 attendees. Like the Midyear, the Annual Meeting offers educational programs on current practice issues, poster and contributed paper sessions, pre-meeting workshops, student programming, and special tracks of educational programming each day. This meeting's smaller size (compared with the Midyear Clinical Meeting) allows prime networking opportunities. The meeting is host to the House of Delegates, the Society's policy-making body. Please refer to the section on ASHP leadership opportunities later in this chapter for a description of the House of Delegates.

ASHP State Affiliate Meetings. These meetings offer the opportunity to become involved in pharmacy practice at a grassroots level and to network more locally. Opportunities for professional growth and development are abundant at this level and include involvement in state government affairs issues and priorities, awareness of concerns unique to the state, opportunities for serving on a committee or as an elected officer, and opportunities for becoming the state affiliate delegate to the ASHP House of Delegates.

The number and content of meetings each state affiliate hosts throughout the year varies; however, this information can be obtained through the ASHP Member and Affiliate Relations division. Most states offer an educational program and some meetings are more extensive, with a House of Delegates meeting taking place.

Special Programs and Conferences

The Competitive Edge. The Competitive Edge program is targeted to pharmacists who obtain and use outcomes data to support pharmacy and therapeutics committee recommendations, develop clinical process tools and deliver pharmaceutical care, support administrative and operational improvement recommendations, and assist an organization in meeting JCAHO and National Committee for Quality Assurance (NCQA) accreditation standards.

Specifically, this program is designed to teach pharmacy's leaders how to gather and use outcomes data to make health-system decisions. At the end of this program, participants are able to evaluate existing outcome studies efficiently and accurately and design simple outcomes studies and use the resulting data to support the formulary decision process, assess the results of a targeted pharmaceutical intervention program such as drug utilization evaluation, support the development and evaluation of clinical services, aid administrative decisions on operational improvement, and assist in meeting JCAHO and NCQA accreditation standards.

Additionally, the program has the following unique components:

- Hands-on: Participants complete an outcomes project for their health system.
- Intimate: Limited class size—one instructor for every eight participants—ensures that attendees receive individual attention.
- Accessible: Between sessions, participants meet regularly (via Internet) with faculty and other students.
- Diverse: The learning experiences are varied (hands-on project experience, workshops, and self-study), making the training interesting and enjoyable.
- Inspiring: Participants have the opportunity to learn from and network with practitioners from across the country.
- CE plus a certificate: Participants earn 42 hours of continuing pharmaceutical education credit from an ACPE-approved provider and a framed certificate of completion.

The program takes place congruently in two different geographic sites. Each site accepts a maximum of 16 participants. Approximately one month before the start of the first session, an applicant is notified of his or her acceptance into the program and receives about 40 hours of pre-training reading material and assignments. Session one takes place simultaneously in two locations. This session is characterized by intensive workshops in which participants review advanced-level concepts in areas such as designing and conducting outcomes research; evaluating published outcomes studies; and applying outcomes data through lecture, case studies, and role play. At this session, each participant identifies a project to conduct in his or her health system.

The time between session one and session two allows the participant to apply what he or she has learned by conducting an outcomes project at the participant's health system. Session two takes place at the same workshop locations and participants report on their project's progress and get feedback from faculty and peers. The completed project is shared with students and faculty from both locations at a special wrap-up session before the ASHP Midyear Clinical Meeting and is featured at a poster session during the meeting.

Qualified participants are practicing pharmacists who already have a fundamental understanding of pharmacoeconomic and outcomes concepts and basic drug information skills. Additional requirements include:

- two years of post-residency practice experience,
- access to clinical data and patients to conduct an outcomes project,
- support of a participant's immediate supervisor, including a commitment to allow him or her to participate in the entire program and complete an outcomes project in the health system,
- access to the Internet, and
- basic knowledge of how to use spreadsheets.

Leadership Conference. The Leadership Conference is sponsored by the ASHP Center on Pharmacy Practice Management and offers pharmacy leaders an opportunity to discuss current trends and challenges in pharmacy practice management. Enrollment for the conference is limited to facilitate interactive sessions. The conference is designed for progressive pharmacy directors and managers, as well as new pharmacy leaders. Information regarding this conference can be obtained on the ASHP Web site or by contacting the ASHP Center on Pharmacy Practice Management.

Pharmacy Leadership Institute. The goal of the Pharmacy Leader-

Home Care

Stanley N. Chamallas, R.Ph., FASHP

Senior Manager Home Infusion Therapy/HME Consulting, Simione Central

Stanley Chamallas develops the marketing program for Simione Central's Home Infusion Therapy/HME division and is a consultant for various clients. He has been in consulting since 1999. After graduating from Northeastern University, Mr. Chamallas went to work at Hermann Hospital in Houston, Texas. While there, Mr. Chamallas got involved with a total parenteral nutrition program and became one of the first pharmacists at Home Health Care of America (HHCA). HHCA later became Caremark, an industry leader in home infusion. He was promoted to Manager of Technical Services at the corporate office and was responsible for developing the bulk compounding process, pharmacy operations policy and procedures, and pharmacy software. He developed standards of practice, hired new pharmacists, and audited field operations. Before moving to Texas, he had worked in the community-based retail environment and feels this experience prepared him for the fast-paced, short-staffed environment of home infusion.

Mr. Chamallas has been active with ASHP, especially the Section of Home Care Practitioners, serving as the Director-at-Large and recently becoming Chair-Elect. He was on the Professional Practice Committee for one year and has been on the Committee for Public Relations and Governmental Affairs for three years, serving as the liaison to the Section of Home Care Practitioners Executive Committee. He serves as a facilitator for the Home Care Section Networking Roundtables at national meetings and has presented at these meetings. He has also published his work with ASHP. He feels these activities have benefited his professional development by providing access to information and interaction with other health care professionals in his field of practice.

Mr. Chamallas recommends that new practitioners interested in home care "join the ASHP Home Care Section and try to become active. Attend networking roundtables and bring questions. Join the Home Care Section Listserv and stay on top of the dialog. There is a tremendous wealth of knowledge being shared." He expresses the importance of taking an active role in communicating the service of pharmacy to legislators.

When Mr. Chamallas hires, he looks for pharmacists with an interest in clinical patient care but with the work ethic to compound intravenous medications or supervise this action as the situation dictates. He emphasizes the importance of flexibility and good interpersonal skills.

ship Institute at the Executive Leadership Center of Boston University is to broaden the business skills, managerial versatility, and the extraordinary leadership demanded of today's directors of health-system pharmacy. The Leadership Institute is targeted to health-system pharmacy directors with five or more years of management experience.

The objectives of this program are to

- develop visionary leaders who can inspire people to make significant contributions and move their organizations forward,
- promote innovative, out-of-the-box thinking,
- energize accomplished managers with new insights, information, and strategies to tackle the challenges of an increasingly complex environment, and
- equip participants for the roles of coach, teacher, motivator, and strategist.

Although the Leadership Institute is not appropriate for a pharmacist in the new practitioner stage of his or her career, it is a resource a new practitioner should keep in mind for the future as his or her career progresses into the management level.

Resources

Online Information Resources. ASHP has developed courses to assist pharmacists in preparation for the Board of Pharmaceutical Specialties (BPS) certification examinations. The completion of these review courses lead to the increased knowledge and skills of pharmacists interested in advanced-level educational programs. Content of these courses is based on the BPS domains, and knowledge areas will be tested on the examinations. The topics have been proportioned according to domains and knowledge area emphasis. More information regarding these courses can be found at www.ashp.org.

Online CE. In an effort to meet members' needs for convenient sources of continuing education, ASHP has placed CE opportunities on the Web. CE articles featured in *AJHP* and virtual symposia can be accessed at www.ashp.org. ASHP's online testing system allows a user to submit a CE test, receive a grade, and get a certificate immediately.

Home Care

Practitioner Spotlight

Donald J. Filibeck, Pharm.D., M.B.A.

Regional Infusion, Pharmacy Manager, Apria Healthcare

Dr. Donald Filibeck is responsible for the day-to-day operations of a $650,000 per month infusion pharmacy operation. The services offered by his department include both infusion and enteral services. He oversees pharmacy, nursing, and customer service, as well as provides clinical support for sales. He is involved in various regional performance improvement groups and corporate committees.

In addition to Dr. Filibeck's responsibilities at Apria Healthcare, he is a surveyor for the Joint Commission on Accreditation of Healthcare Organizations. In this position, he conducts home care pharmacy surveys. He is also a member of the Parenteral Compounding Expert Committee, United States Pharmacopeia.

Following graduation from pharmacy school, Dr. Filibeck practiced for six years in hospital pharmacy. He was involved in direct patient care, clinical support, and oversight of the operations and personnel in the intravenous room. He left the hospital as an assistant director and began his career in home care. He has had thirteen years of experience in home care with varying levels of responsibility, including positions with regional pharmacy support of multisite locations. He completed a Masters of Business Administration (M.B.A.) degree ten years after graduating with his Pharm.D. degree. He has found his M.B.A. to be very beneficial as it provides the business insight that is necessary today.

Dr. Filibeck has been involved with ASHP primarily through activity in the Section of Home Care Practitioners. He has served as the Director-at-Large and the Chair of the section and was involved in the development of the Home Care Competency Assessment Tool. He has also been involved in the creation of ASHP publications. Dr. Filibeck states, "I have been extremely impressed by the people I have met through ASHP. The staff is excellent. It has allowed me to meet individuals of prominence in the profession that I do not feel I would have met without the involvement in ASHP."

When hiring, he looks for someone with a good clinical background along with a willingness to learn. Experience in pharmacokinetics and nutrition is also advantageous. Dr. Filibeck concludes, "Take advantage of every opportunity. Explore options. Continue to educate yourself by taking courses and attending continuing education programs that not only broaden your pharmacy knowledge, but also may be centered on other areas, such as computers. Constantly ask 'why?'"

Print Publications

Clinical Skills Program. This comprehensive, multifaceted clinical skills program includes instructional self-study modules, workshops, computer-assisted learning, and resource texts. The core of the program consists of three series of modules designed to help a practitioner develop problem-solving skills in providing patient-specific pharmacotherapy and drug information.

Self-Study Courses. ASHP offers various self-study products, including *Concepts in Clinical Pharmacokinetics* and *Concepts in Immunology and Immunotherapeutics*. These self-study courses allow practitioners to learn at their own pace and to earn continuing education.

***American Journal of Health-System Pharmacy* (*AJHP*).** *AJHP* is the official journal of the society, covering all aspects of health-system pharmacy from health care management to progressive drug therapy. *AJHP* is read by more health-system pharmacists than any other pharmacy publication. The journal is distributed twice a month and contains articles on practice and products, professional practice standards, primers and guidelines, drug and drug therapy reviews, the latest health care Web sites, book reviews, career development information, job listings, current literature, and more. In addition, *AJHP* features special interest articles exploring issues unique to particular practice settings or practice management. A subscription to *AJHP* is included in the society's membership dues.

Leadership Opportunities and Development

Board of Directors. The governing body of ASHP, the Board of Directors, is responsible for the effective administration and management of the society. The Board meets four times per year and recommends professional policies to the House of Delegates for ratification. It is responsible for developing a budget, financial controls, and investment programs that ensure continued growth and stability. Members of the Board are elected by ASHP's active members on an at-large basis.

House of Delegates. The highlight of the Annual Meeting is the ASHP House of Delegates, the society's policy-making body. The House of Delegates includes state delegates, members of the ASHP Board of Directors, ASHP past presidents, fraternal representation, chairs of the sections, and student delegates. The delegates are at the center of ASHP's professional policy development and approval process. The delegates attend regional delegate conferences to educate and inform them of topical professional policy issues. Delegates and all attendees can also participate in the open hearings conducted at the Annual Meeting and the Midyear Clinical Meeting. To be a member of the House of Delegates, you must be an ASHP member. Delegate elections are administered by your ASHP state affiliate.

Advisory Groups, Councils, Commissions, and Committees. ASHP's five councils—Administrative, Educational, Legal and Public, Organizational, and Professional Affairs—handle some of the society's most important policy functions. The councils serve ASHP in policy development and advisory capacities. In addition, a number of ASHP advisory groups, commissions, and committees serve the organization. These groups make recommendations that guide the organization and the profession. Appointments to these bodies typically occur through the society's elected president. Let the president or members of ASHP's staff know if you are interested in such an appointment.

Other Ways to Get Involved with ASHP

Professional Practice and Scientific Affairs. A major commitment of ASHP is the development of therapeutic position statements, which are published in *AJHP* and incorporated into the annual update of *Best Practices for Health-System Pharmacy*. These ASHP Statements, Guidelines, and Therapeutics Guidelines comprise the most complete body of continually updated advice available on practice in hospitals and other health systems. ASHP members develop these professional documents. Take advantage of opportunities to draft, review, and comment on these important documents.

Reviewers and Contributors. Another highly visible way to get involved in ASHP is by volunteering to serve as a reviewer or contributor for *AJHP*. Your contribution could take the form of an editorial, clinical review, therapy update, report, or commentary.

Meeting Programming Associates. Your knowledge is needed to guide the educational programming for the Midyear Clinical and Annual Meetings. Perhaps you have the expertise necessary to plan an educational program, review a paper submitted for presentation at a national meeting, present a pearl session, lead a roundtable discussion, or moderate an educational session. Contact the ASHP Educational Services Division to find out how you might get more involved in this role.

Member Recruiter. Encourage your colleagues to become ASHP members and reap the rewards. Contact ASHP for a supply of membership applications, and take it from there. You may receive a variety of rewards and recognition for introducing other practitioners to ASHP.

State Society Leadership. ASHP encourages member involvement with state affiliates. Various opportunities exist on the state level for involvement and leadership development with an affiliated society. Contact ASHP's Member and Affiliate Relations Division to find out who your state affiliate contact person is and explore the opportunities available on a more local level.

Access to ASHP Information and Staff

We have outlined numerous ways for new practitioners to become more actively involved with ASHP and the pharmacy profession in general. For assistance in this endeavor, please contact ASHP for additional information and guidance. The ASHP Web site (www.ashp.org) offers a wealth of information about ASHP activities and opportunities. Additionally, you may contact ASHP staff for information at the numbers on pages 97 and 98.

Getting Involved with Legislative Issues

The ASHP Government Affairs division uses grassroots communications and political action activities to advocate ASHP policy and positions before federal and state policymakers and the courts. This group works to empower the membership to work in partnership with ASHP and its state affiliates to achieve public policy that helps people make the best use of medicines.

This division coordinates and supports the following programs and activities:

- works with other national pharmacy organizations to advocate coverage of pharmacists' patient care services,
- analyzes legislative and regulatory proposals and offers amendments and other changes where necessary,
- advocates incorporation of ASHP policy in federal and state legislation and regulation,
- provides testimony, statements, and written comments to congressional committees and federal and state agencies,

Contacting ASHP

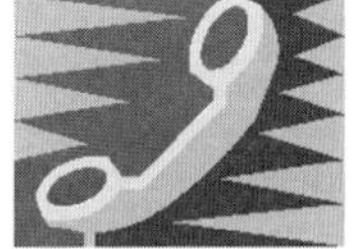

ASHP Main Phone Number (301) 657-3000
(www.ashp.org)

For information on .... Call this extension

Accreditation Services Division (ASD) / Residency Programs x1251
(asd@ashp.org)

Administration, Technology, and Information Systems x1300

American Journal of Health-System Pharmacy (AJHP) x1200
(ajhp@ashp.org)

ASHP Research and Education Foundation x1447
(Foundation@ashp.org)

ASHP Staff .... (Info@ashp.org)

Brochure Request Line x1320

Career Development Service (CDS) x1289

Career Opportunities in *AJHP* x1288

Center on Patient Safety x1270

Center on Pharmacy Practice Management x1350

Continuing Education Self-Study Programs x1281

Customer Service x1524
(Custserv@ashp.org)

Drug Information Databases
(*IPA*, *AHFS Drug Information*, Online & CD-ROM products) x1254

Educational Services Division (ESD) x1281
(educserv@ashp.org)

Government Affairs Division (GAD) x1306
(gad@ashp.org)

Membership .... (membership@ashp.org)

Member and Affiliate Relations (MAR) x1289

Personnel Placement Service (PPS) x1344

continued next page

Pharmacy Student Forum x1289
(Students@ashp.org)

Professional Practice and Scientific Affairs Division (PPSAD) x1282

Publications, Software, and Videotapes x1202

Public Relations x1224

Section of Clinical Specialists x1266
(Clinspec@ashp.org)

Section of Home Care Practitioners x1400
(Homecare@ashp.org)

State Affiliates x1289
(Chapters@ashp.org)

Technicians x1338

ASHP Fax Numbers

Publication and Product Orders 800-665-ASHP (x2747)

International Fax Orders 301-657-1215

Fax-on-Demand 301-664-8888

- generates ASHP member and constituent response on key issues with a Grassroots Contact System,
- administers a Political Action Committee that back candidates who are supportive of health-system pharmacy's mission and leadership agenda,
- plans educational programs at meetings, as well as letter writing campaigns, generates volunteer involvement, and aids in member retention and recruitment,
- hosts a Legislative Day to engage ASHP policy development volunteers in the advocacy process,
- participates in joint activities with other pharmacy organizations at the National Conference of State Legislatures that support ASHP and state affiliate legislative and regulatory agenda,

- writes issue papers that serve as brief background for policymakers to formulate a position, and

- generates monthly issue summaries to update the membership on key state and federal issues impacting pharmacy.

The ASHP Government Affairs Division is instrumental in keeping ASHP members informed of legislative happenings on national and state levels. Key information updates are routinely posted on the ASHP Web site and distributed through the Grassroots Contact System. A society member may sign up for the Grassroots Contact System by contacting the Government Affairs Division.

Contacting Members of Congress

Legislators and their staff affirm that one of the most effective ways to gain their attention is through individual letters composed and sent by constituents. The goal of writing letters to a member of Congress is to increase the member's awareness of an issue pertaining to pharmacy practice. It is important to define clearly the issue you are writing about, how this issue affects pharmacy practice, and what impact this issue has on patient care and/or pharmacists' abilities to maintain patient care service.

Do not forget in writing letters to members of Congress how little experience the recipient may have with the patient care services of pharmacists. In many cases, the only contact they may have had with a pharmacist is in picking up a prescription. Unless individuals have a more serious or chronic condition, their interaction with a pharmacist does not go beyond this low level of patient care. Each communication you have about an issue must begin by confirming that the individual truly understands the role of the pharmacist in drug therapy management.

ASHP, through its Web site and the Grassroots Contact System, keeps members informed of critical moments in the legislative process when a targeted message must be sent to your representatives in Congress. The initial letter should merely introduce the problem and invite the Congressperson to contact you as a resource for understanding how this problem affects constituents. If, at any time, you need assistance in composing a letter for your member of Congress, contact the Government Affairs Division for assistance.

Building Relationships with Congressional Staff

Members of Congress rely heavily on the expertise of their staff when making public policy decisions, making staff a critical point of contact in the legislative process. Staff track bills in Congress, study issues emerging in society, and make recommendations to their bosses. Staff often control who or what gets to the legislator and "color" the perception of a person or an idea. For these and other reasons, building a good relationship with congressional staff makes good sense.

A legislator's personal staff is made up of people who handle legislation, office operations, new media inquiries, and voter inquiries, as well as scheduling requests from anyone wanting time with the legislator, including constituents, trade groups, reporters, and others. As a voting constituent and a member of ASHP's Grassroots Contact System, you will typically make contact with the legislator's legislative and scheduling staff. The legislative staff ASHP frequently contacts includes legislative assistants who handle health care issues. It is important to make this distinction because staff specialize in a variety of public policy subjects. Legislative assistants manage issues, do research, analyze reports and legislation, and draft legislative proposals. They advise the legislator on what actions should be taken and whether to support or oppose a bill that is up for a vote. A well-prepared and thoughtful letter is likely to be passed on to the legislator or very influential staffers.

Letters and phone calls from constituents may be the most important source of information to a congressional office. About 75% of congressional offices in a recent survey rank information from constituents more important than any other source of information.Your thoughts count more than government reports, news media stories, and information provided by interest groups, finds a poll by Peter D. Hart Research Associates in Washington, D.C. Congressional offices are impressed by letters that show that the writer put a good deal of thought into the writing and that he or she is knowledgeable about the subject. Indeed, a one-page letter from a constituent tells legislators that between 20 and 300 people in the district likely feel the same way, estimates a senior staffer in a post-survey interview.

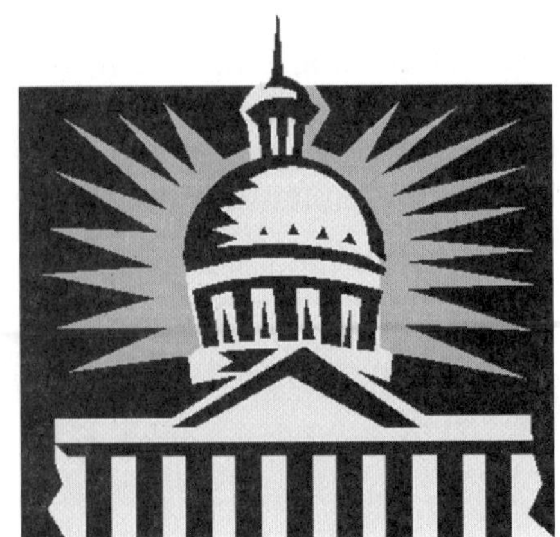

It is important to ASHP advocacy efforts that you work with

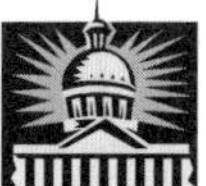

your legislators and their staff. You have the opportunity to educate senators, representatives, and their staffs about the work you do and what they need to do to improve patient care. Since you are a voting constituent, legislators and staff care what you think and want to learn about what their people do for the community; educate them about your job and the patients you serve.

To set up a meeting with your legislator or a staff member, contact your legislator's home office and ask to speak to the scheduler. Introduce yourself to your representative and senators when they are home for the weekend or during a congressional recess. They return home regularly to interact with constituents. Congress adjourns periodically throughout the year (over Easter, during August, and just before Thanksgiving). Consider inviting your members of Congress and their staff on a tour of your practice site. Should you ever visit the Washington, D.C. area, please let ASHP help set up appointments for you with your representatives and senators in their personal offices. Complete contact information for your members of Congress can be found on the Project Vote Smart Web site at www.vote-smart.org. You may also check out www.congress.org to determine who your representatives are. Otherwise, call ASHP's Government Affairs Division at (301) 657-3000 extension 1306, for phone numbers and addresses or to express any questions or concerns you may have.

Preparing for a Meeting with Members of Congress

The following points are important to consider as you prepare to meet face-to-face with a legislator or staff member:

- *Plan your visit carefully.* Be clear about what it is you want to achieve. Determine in advance whether you will be meeting with your elected official or a staff person. Know the committees of which your representative or senator is a member.
- *Make an appointment.* Contact the scheduler for your member of Congress. Explain that you are a health-system pharmacist and a constituent. The scheduler will ask for the purpose of the meeting. It is easier for congressional staff to arrange a meeting if they know what you wish to discuss and your relationship to the official.
- *Be prepared.* Whenever possible, bring to the meeting information and materials supporting your position. Members are required to take positions on many different issues. In some instances, a member may lack important details about the pros and cons of a particular matter. It is, therefore, helpful to provide information and examples

continued next page

that demonstrate clearly the impact or benefits associated with a particular issue or piece of legislation. But don't get technical with your information. The legislator is not a pharmacist and is not familiar with some of the language commonly used in the profession.

- *Be prompt and patient.* When it is time to meet with your legislator, be punctual and patient. It is not uncommon for him or her to be late, or to have a meeting interrupted, due to the legislator's crowded schedule. If interruptions do occur, be flexible; and if the opportunity presents itself, continue your meeting with a member's staff. A typical meeting with a constituent lasts about ten to fifteen minutes.
- *Be sure to budget your time.* Make sure you have enough time to ask the questions you want answered or request the action you want the lawmaker to take.
- *Be political.* Members of Congress want to represent the best interests of their district or state. Whenever possible, demonstrate the connection between what you are requesting and how that will impact others in your district or state. Remember that all politics is local.
- *Be responsive.* Be prepared to answer questions or provide additional information, in the event the member expresses interest or asks questions. Follow up the meeting with a thank-you letter that outlines the different points covered during the meeting, and send along any additional information and material requested. You can call ASHP's Government Affairs Division for this information or gather information from your work.
- *Show your representatives what you do.* Maybe your meeting will follow a brief tour of your practice facility. Legislators are interested in seeing what their constituents do for the community. You and your colleagues should show them around your patient care areas and demonstrate to them the expanded role of pharmacists. Invite the health system's public relations staff to join you and take pictures. After the tour, sit down with them in your office and briefly discuss one or two health policy issues that affect your practice. Be sure to follow up with them by sending any photographs, news releases, or stories that my have come out of the visit. Be sure to send a copy to ASHP's Government Affairs Division.
- *Do not threaten!* Do not threaten to withhold your vote and do not discuss campaign contributions. These points are highly unproductive, and telling your legislators you contributed to their campaigns is illegal.

The following points are important to note when writing a letter to your member of Congress:

Properly address your legislators. When writing to a member of Congress, address your letter to "The Honorable John Smith" or "Dear Senator Smith" or "Dear Representative Smith," whatever the case may be. Verify the address and spelling of the name of your representative and senators.

Keep your message brief and to the point. Discuss only one issue, and try to keep the letter to one page. Make it clear that you are a voting constituent who lives in the representative's district or your senator's state. Your ideas and recommendations count. State the purpose of your letter in the first paragraph.

If your letter pertains to a specific piece of legislation, identify it according to bill number. For example, H.R. 4860 refers to a bill before the House of Representatives, and S. 2772 to a bill before the Senate. ASHP provides you with this information in its monthly Issue Summaries. Using the bill number in your letters will help congressional staffers identify the bill you're referring to and will eliminate any confusion.

Discuss the issue in relation to what is happening at home. Legislators and staffers want to know what is going on at home. They are in Washington to represent you, and they can do their job better if you tell them what you need. Using real life examples helps clarify your concerns. For instance, you might say that it is important that Medicare have an outpatient prescription drug benefit because some of your elderly patients are not properly taking their medications. You will drive home your point if you discuss how Mrs. Johnson fills her 30-day supply of Prilosec only once every three months because she cannot afford more. By taking only a third of her doctor's prescribed dose, she is risking a serious health problem.

Be the concerned citizen that you are. You are more effective as a concerned citizen than as a member of a lobbying effort. A good letter that is honest and that genuinely reflects your concerns is taken very seriously. It is all right to mention you are a member of ASHP, but don't let your letter look like it was prompted by the society's Legislative Action Alert.

Provide contact information in your letter. Your letter should contain your return address and telephone number so your representatives or staff may follow up with you.

References and Resources

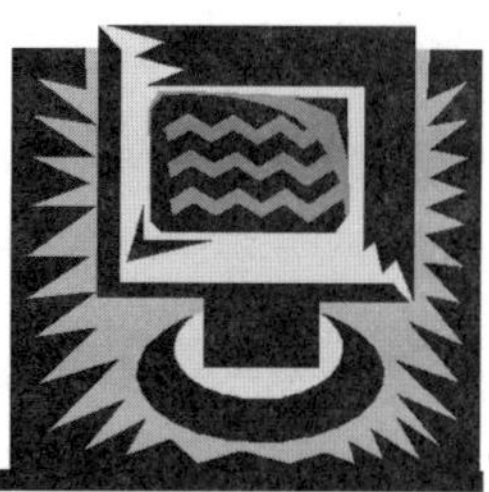

Online References

http://www.ashp.org/students/pdb2001.pdf

http://www.ashp.org/public/public_relations/handouts/ashpfact.html References Chapter 8

http://www.ashp.org/public/meetings/annual/index.html

http://www.ashp.org/public/meetings/midyear/mcm2001/index.html

http://www.ashp.org/public/news/newsletters/student/1998/fall98/residency.html

http://www.ashp.org/public/meetings/leader/

http://www.ashp.org/public/meetings/ceos.html

http://www.ashp.org/public/ceonline/index.html

http://www.ashp.org/oncology/

http://www.ashp.org/practicemanagement/leadership2001.html

http://www.ashp.org/public/proad/mission.html

http://www.ashp.org/public/proad/letter.html

http://www.ashp.org/public/proad/meeting.html

http://www.ashp.org/public/proad/relationships.html

http://www.ashp.org/public/news/breaking/ShowArticle.cfm?id=2000

http://www.ashp.org/clinical/oncology_review.html

http://www.ashp.org/clinical/psych_review.html

http://www.ashp.org/public/proad/compensation/

http://www.ashp.org/public/rtp

Additional References

"Professional Development: Residencies, The ASHP Midyear Clinical Meeting, and More...." Katherine P. Smith, Pharm.D.; Edited by Sandra L. Baldinger, Pharm.D., M.S. (ASHP 2000)

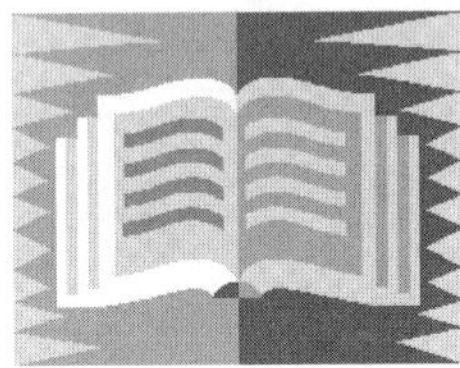

"At Your Service: ASHP Membership Benefits and Opportunities" brochure (ASHP)

"Health-System Pharmacists Do More Than Fill Prescriptions" brochure (ASHP)

"Shall I Study Pharmacy?" brochure (American College of Apothecaries, Academy of Managed Care Pharmacy, American Pharmaceutical Association, American Society of Consultant Pharmacists, American Society of Health-System Pharmacists, National Association of Boards of Pharmacy, National Association of Chain Drug Stores, Pharmaceutical Research and Manufacturers of America)

"Why Do I Need a Hospital Pharmacist?" brochure (ASHP)

"Pharmacy Residencies" brochure (ASHP)